THE MISSION OF MAYA AND METHUSELAH

A Medical Guide for Aging in Place

Karen Marie Humphreys

MD, FRCPC INTERNAL MEDICINE SPECIALIST

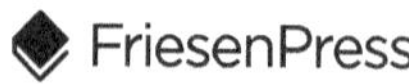

One Printers Way
Altona, MB R0G 0B0
Canada

www.friesenpress.com

ISBN
978-1-03-915572-5 (Hardcover)
978-1-03-915571-8 (Paperback)
978-1-03-915573-2 (eBook)

1. MED032000 MEDICAL, GERIATRICS

Distributed to the trade by The Ingram Book Company

TABLE OF CONTENTS

v   Dedication

1   Introduction

19   Chapter 1: Frailty Definitions and Details

33   Chapter 2: Current Health Care Limitations as the
         Population Ages

43   Chapter 3: Key Essentials for Optimal Aging

50   Chapter 4: Essentials of Exercise Prescriptions and
         Cardiac Rehabilitation

68   Chapter 5: Essentials of Respiratory Rehabilitation Programs

83   Chapter 6: Essentials of Low Resistance Weight Training

91   Chapter 7: Balance and Brain Training for Adults of All Ages

102   Chapter 8: Combining Routines and Activity Plans from
         Chapters 4-7

114   Chapter 9: Preparation for Action in the Fifties—Maya and Her
         Mother Maria

131   Chapter 10: Preparation for Action in the Sixties—
         Deborah's Case

141   Chapter 11: Preparation for Action in the Seventies

154   Chapter 12: Preparation for Action in the Eighties

162   Chapter 13: Preparation for Action at Ninety-Plus Years

170   Chapter 14: Essentials of Home Assessment and Allied Health
         Professional Input

175   Chapter 15: Need/Role for Comprehensive Geriatric Assessments

183   Chapter 16: The Butterfly and the Lobster

187   Chapter 17: Determining Your Motivation for Change –
         Karen's Story

195   Chapter 18: Wish List for the Future

204   Chapter 19: Conclusions

211   Bibliography

DEDICATION

This book is dedicated to my younger sister, Lisa, who tragically passed away in May 2020, during the COVID-19 pandemic. Her death might have been preventable had she not experienced mental health issues, marginalization, and inequality secondary to her socioeconomic status. She was a writer and is part of the reason for me writing this book.

"Lisa, I am so sorry Kathy and I will not get the opportunity to grow old together. Rest in peace, Sis!" —Karen

INTRODUCTION

Very few of us look forward to aging. As we embark upon the latter third of our lives, we are hopeful that our living situation and circumstances will afford us a good quality and reasonable quantity of life. Unfortunately, the COVID-19 pandemic unearthed many significant health-care crises in primary care, hospital care and long-term care facilities in Canada and abroad. The latter has been eloquently discussed in André Picard's book *Neglected No More*, where he thoroughly speaks of the current long-term care crisis and the proposed interventions required to fix these issues.[1]

Many of the long-term care residents exhibit frailty, which contributes to poor outcomes. While frailty will accelerate our need for more in-depth personal care as we age, frailty itself is not a normal part of aging. Frailty is a precursor to many negative outcomes, including but not exclusive to falls, physical and cognitive decline, hospitalizations, worse outcomes with surgeries, and an overall increase in disabilities. All of these processes could contribute to acute care hospitalization or long-term care institutionalization and even a higher mortality rate. There are many complicated physiologic aging changes that are beyond the scope of this book that contribute to the development of frailty. Some of these processes happen whether we want them to, or not. Some of the processes could be within an individual's control, which is the topic upon which I will focus. These general aging systemic transitions are best reviewed with clinicians who are experts in the field of geriatrics. What we all need to acknowledge, however, is that frailty can and should be prevented in situations where this is possible. Otherwise, the unintended result will be increased vulnerability to almost any stressor, which is a trigger for adverse health-care outcomes and increased mortality.

As an expert in adult medicine, I know that there are more than

---

1   Picard, André. *Neglected No More: The Urgent Need to Improve the Lives of Canadian Elders in the Wake of a Pandemic.* Penguin Random House, March 2021.

sixty assessment tools available to detect frailty in older populations. Some of these rely on paper or computerized scoring systems that assess an individual's level of risk. Some of these frailty scores are used on a regular basis during geriatric assessments. Sometimes the government will utilize these scoring systems during census data collection to review our aging society. These agencies use the data to denote frailty in the general population or use the frailty data to prioritize care for vulnerable clients within the health care system.

Frailty exists on a spectrum of functional robustness to the other extreme, which is failure to thrive/preterminal status (one foot in the grave, so to speak).

Frailty can also be associated with a perceived decreased quality of life, along with an increased need for physical, emotional, and psychological support. As we age, most of us want to carry on with a good quality of life, free of suffering, pain, discomfort, while continuing to have a purpose and finding pleasure in our day-to-day activities. Frailty takes away a great deal of our independence. For generations, people have become old and frail with very few exceptions.

Overall, our societal norms expect people to age and decrease activities, but this should not be encouraged. As I carry on with my occupation of adult medicine specialist (Internal Medicine), I am constantly reminded (in hours of meetings each week) of how fragile and increasingly dysfunctional, our health care system is. At this point in time, the current governments and ministries are reviewing all types of health care in many jurisdictions. In Canada, everyone knows the current system is overwhelmed and is already unable to keep up with the demands that an increasingly older and frail population places on the entire health care system. Meetings occur daily in almost every facility, trying to extinguish the flames of overcapacity, due in part to a lack of long-term care home placement beds, a lack of acute care hospital beds, and a loss of human resources that have been accentuated with a global pandemic, that has not been eradicated as yet. Governments, ministries, health authorities, and care facilities are in reactive or crisis mode. Very few meetings look past the next day, week, month, or year. But what is waiting for us is far more concerning.

We are getting older as a society. We have a lack of trained talent working in almost every industry. We have a large burden of inflation and many families struggle without at least two incomes. We also have a devasting lack of primary care, which makes medical assessments of all ages of our population less than ideal. In addition, our aging population has not always valued fitness as a preventative strategy for disease or frailty prevention. This is combined with the fact that generationally, we are not always willing or financially able to care for older relatives. We are seeing, with increasing frequency, that our own adult children have financial instability and stay in the parental home for an extended period due to finance constraints, higher levels of inflation and the high price of education and housing. This makes for a very tenuous situation when planning any family-centric options for an older relative requiring care in the family home. There often is not enough physical space or family finances for this to be a feasible option. We must then rely on these seniors to fend for themselves. There are still many cultures that value the privilege of looking after their elders. But it is getting more and more difficult to sustain these traditions. Society believes and accepts that aging and becoming weak or frail is expected. I am here to tell you it is not.

As our population ages, if we don't change *how* we age with regards to our finances, fitness, and functionality, there will be an even larger demand for access to long-term care *without* the availability of these resources (available space and staff to manage increased long-term bed capacity) to provide that care. If we think this is bad now, if we wait for another ten years for the population to further age, it will become unmanageable.

In this book, I will talk about frailty in our Canadian population, but this will apply to many other countries as well. I will also explore the things individuals can do in their latter third of life to help prevent frailty and the potentially negative outcomes associated with it. Time is of the essence! Every workday, I see elderly patients who get some mode of therapy to try and address the frailty. There never seems to be any sustained improvement as the "prescription for activity" is one that is basic and often, is not continued by family or reinforced in the community. I also note that due to a severe lack of community resources, the plan rarely incorporates firm goals or long-term expectations for the older adult to progress or increase their fitness level. As a health care professional, I see the same clients being admitted to hospital repeatedly, especially in their last year of life, and with each hospitalization, there is an additional stepwise further functional decline. This stepwise deconditioning continues until they eventually experience the "celestial discharge."

Are we too late in most of these hospitalized cases? I believe so when it comes to acutely admitted hospitalized elders. By the time frailty is identified in a hospitalized senior, very little can reverse the frailty score and/or the negative outcomes associated with this frail status.

Therefore, frailty concerns must be addressed at the individual, family, and primary care level before hospitalization or institutionalization, in order to improve fitness and functionality as we get older.

With this book, I hope to enlighten seniors and their family members about the perils of frailty and give some guidance on prevention. I also wish to focus on what clients, family members, and concerned friends or citizens can to help negotiate this fragile time of lack of access to primary care for all adult Canadians.

This book is about the mission of Maya and Methuselah, the youngest and the oldest fictional clients used in the clinical scenarios. Maya's name was inspired by the legend of Maya Angelou, who was an iconic elderly American poet, aging, and civil rights activist. Her work life was lengthy, over many decades. She was renowned for her ability to actively tour as a guest speaker, up until her eight decade of life. She was an inspiration to many people, but particularly women of colour. She was a revered as a respected spokesperson for all people of her ethnicity.

Her book *And Still I Rise* was a great illustration of a Black woman's life experiences and subsequent resilience. It's an excellent poem for every person, regardless of ethnicity, gender, sexuality, nationality, or socioeconomic status. It is a poem promoting humans to enhance progress, and continue to move forward, regardless of what life has in store for us and the perceived life issues.[2]

---

2   Angelou, Maya. And Still I Rise. Random House.

Excerpt from: "Still I Rise" by Maya Angelou

Did you want to see me broken?
Bowed head and lowered eyes?
Shoulders falling down like teardrops,
Weakened by my soulful cries?

Does my haughtiness offend you?
Don't you take it awful hard
'Cause I laugh like I've got gold mines
Diggin' in my own backyard.

You may shoot me with your words,
You may cut me with your eyes,
You may kill me with your hatefulness,
But still, like air, I'll rise.

......

I am the dream and the hope of the slave.
I rise
I rise
I rise.

The final fictional client is named Methuselah. Unlike the biblical Methuselah, this gentleman was not 969 years of age before he died. He was a robust man until his ninety-second year, when illness and misfortune rapidly bounced him out of the robust category and into the very frail category. Once known for his physical activities (dancing), persistence, wisdom, and problem-solving skills, his illness rendered him incapacitated from a physical, emotional, psychological, and financial standpoint. The persona of Methuselah is based on my knowledge of one exceptional nonagenarian in my life, who rapidly declined due to unforeseen medical events and illness.

While these two characters are the youngest and the oldest of the clients in my clinical scenarios, each fictional client is based on my interactions with real-life people throughout my many years of client interactions and acquaintances. I use these client scenarios as examples to discuss and illustrate complicated latter-life planning, that encompasses general care and recommendations, exercise prescriptions, brain training and socialization, financial planning, and advocacy suggestions for these clients and their families. The concepts discussed in each scenario may apply to many people in the similar age groups within the general population. I encourage advocacy for elder care from all interested individuals and corporations in the community. I will try to elaborate on how adult Canadians can navigate this current dysfunctional health care system as we age, with or without known medical conditions or documented ailments.

The book is merely a jumping off point to initiate discussions regarding problem solving with the ultimate goal to improve global elder care as soon as possible.

We are currently in a primary care crisis in Canada and *many* other countries. There are general health and screening guidelines that caregivers should ensure are reviewed for each individual client/patient. At one point in my own life, when I didn't have a primary care provider, I was denied a screening mammogram, as I did not have a primary care provider to follow up on the results. As a physician, I had to advocate for myself to get this screening test done. I had to go through various levels of managers to get a mammogram in my mid-fifties. It was only when I told them that I was a physician and would go to the media if I wasn't allowed to book this necessary screening test, that I was allowed to use a co-worker's name to receive the mammogram results. It donned on me, at that point in my life, how broken our healthcare system is. I'm fortunate to have had colleagues bail me out, but I wondered how many other women were being denied basic cancer screening tests because they didn't have a dedicated primary care provider? This is embarrassingly common in my province and in most of Canada.

I could advocate for myself, due to my knowledge of the healthcare system and the hierarchical layers. My largest gripe with the current status of health care is that there is often limited accountability at every level of the hierarchy, and often I wonder if anyone really cares about the patients in our society.

I know the system is broken and on the verge of collapse. Who is looking out for our society members who have no current access to primary care? All provincial governments and the federal government are aware of the crisis. The premiers and health ministers are currently in talks to get more funding from the federal government. However, I have not seen any universal robust plan to increase global access to primary care on a large (provincial/urban/rural/remote) scale. After years of poor planning across the entire country and a global pandemic that has burnt out almost every essential worker in every industry, we are now scrambling to find suitably trained professionals. These professionals require anywhere between two and ten years of training. We are all praying that this massive gap is filled before the entire system collapses. There are options for recruiting professionals from other jurisdictions, but these resources are also limited and the gap in training enough professionals is an issue created decades ago.

This book aims to give some guidance to those of you struggling to find primary health care. I implore every one of you to start advocating now for yourselves and your elders in order to prevent illnesses that are easily screened for by having a primary care provider. It is a shame when treatable conditions such as early-stage cancers, hypertension, diabetes, chronic kidney disease, heart disease, and cerebral vascular disease are not found until they are too far gone or there has already been end organ damage. All because of a lack of access to primary health care. And while primary health care is critically absent in many parts of the world, access to geriatricians for the aging populations in many countries like Canada is profoundly limited.[3] This is quite an unstable paradox, as the baby boomer generation slowly gets older every year.

---

3   Nathan Stall, "Who Will Care for Canada's Seniors?" healthy debate, August 8, 2013, https://healthydebate.ca/2013/08/topic/community-long-term-care/who-will-care-for-canadas-seniors/#:~:text=All%20in%20all%2C%20there%20are%20approximately%20325%20full-time,medicine%20serving%20a%20population%20of%202.0%20million%20seniors.

Total number & number/100,000 population by province 2019

Province/Territory	Geriatric Physicians	Physicians per 100,000 Population
Newfoundland/Labrador	1	0.2
Prince Edward Island	1	0.6
Nova Scotia	11	1.1
New Brunswick	7	0.9
Quebec	83	0.0
Ontario	126	0.9
Manitoba	6	0.4
Saskatchewan	1	0.1
Alberta	20	0.5
British Columbia	48	1.0
Territories	0	0.0
Canada	304	0.8

2019 CMA Masterfile 7 Number/100,000 population, 2019[4]

Geriatricians primarily see the most frail and vulnerable elderly clients in the community, but most of the referrals are generated by practitioners for hospitalized clients or those community clients who have access to some member of the health care team. But this volume of seniors seeking out geriatric consultations is just the tip of the iceberg. There are many more clients, living in unsafe home situations, who do not have access to any care. They exist in their own homes, not always safe to cook, predisposed to falling, and suffering from general ill health that nobody notices until it's very late in the process. This is usually when a wellness check or concerned community member contacts authorities, or the senior has a fall or other hospital presentation.

Do you know someone in your life who lives like this? If so, what have you done to reach out to assist this individual? While I think we all know someone in this situation, many of us feel that we would be "intruding" if we step in or enquire about their situation. We are now at

---

4   "Geriatric Medicine Profile," Canadian Medical Association, accessed August 21, 2022, https://www.cma.ca/sites/default/files/2019-01/geriatric-e.pdf.

a time in history with an all-time low in access to primary health care, a broken safety net for timely access to ambulance services and emergency room care (without extensive delays) that requires us as a community to step up and try to offer some assistance if we can do so.

There aren't enough geriatricians to support our growing aging population. Therefore, primary care providers, specialists, allied health professionals, clinic staff, families, and community members must *all* take a stand in advocating for better eldercare today.

It all starts with education of the general public, which is the purpose of this book.

There are distinct physiological and pathological changes of aging that we must understand, identify, diagnose, and treat, if the disease entity is amenable to treatment. This requires access to primary health care.

There are some estimates that in British Columbia up to 900,000+ patients are without a primary care provider. This concerns me on several fronts. For example, one of my close acquaintances, who is a newly diagnosed diabetic and gets her medications from the walk-in clinic in her community, does not have a consistent care giver for longitudinal follow up with her repeat visits. While she does get her medications refilled and quarterly diabetic blood work organized, those clinicians, who have only seen her on one occasion, are unable to see that she has the start of dementia. If taken out of her own home, she's not able to manage. While she says that she walks on a regular basis, it's evident that she hasn't been walking and has no real activity tolerance. Her sons have asked her not to drive long distances, and she has reluctantly complied with that request. Her family has witnessed that when she is in any unfamiliar environment, she is now easily flustered, is unable to problem solve, and gets very agitated.

I know many adults in their forties and fifties who don't have a primary care provider, but they feel well and still believe they are invincible. These individuals have not thought about checking their own blood pressure, even if the opportunity presents itself. They're not usually curious enough to go out and buy a blood pressure machine, because until they're diagnosed with an illness or disease, people in this age group simply believe they are healthy! Does this sound familiar?

From my perspective as an adult medicine specialist, simple actions—like checking your blood pressure on a regular basis—can help prevent potentially devastating consequences of hypertension-related diseases, including heart attack, stroke, vision impairment, and chronic kidney disease. Therefore, my general medical recommendations regarding health in each of the scenarios in this book will include some self-initiated assessments with regards to things like monitoring your own blood pressure or arranging screening general health exams. This is so important, especially if you are one of the 900,000+ British Columbians without a primary care provider. I will also point you toward available websites that also support these initiatives. Again, the primary care crisis is not exclusive to Canada, as many other countries and jurisdictions have the same primary care resource deficiency.

Another important concept explored in this book is the financial truth that aging can be costly. Medication requirements and disease diagnoses increase as we age. There is an abundance of evidence in the medical literature that suggests that single illnesses such as diabetes, heart disease, and hypertension will require the use of several categories of medications for additive beneficial effects. There has been a shift in study protocols to now include adults in their eighties and nineties in studies, because the population is successfully getting older and living longer with treatments derived from studies over the last three to four decades.

This successful living longer with chronic diseases results in the need for advanced financial planning to cover the costs as we age. However, this planning must be done *before* clients are diagnosed with illnesses or put on medications. In the insurance industry, pre-existing disease diagnoses often render a client uninsurable. This means that there will need to be a financial plan in place for medication costs, long-term care, coverage during hospitalization for critical illness, or loss of employment. If these unfortunate scenarios are planned for in a timely manner, when the cost of insurance products is still affordable, these individuals can be reassured that the financial impact of the care needs are lessened. In other words, if you choose not to plan for these events when you're younger, then you or your family must bear the financial burden as you age. This further adds to the stress associated of aging. One day, you may need to self-fund for medications, accommodation needs, nursing care interventions, live-in assistance, and/or moving to a long-term care facility.

There is an incredible amount of planning that needs to be looked at, starting in our forties and fifties, in order to prepare for our last ten to fifteen years of existence. At the current time, the Canada Health Act doesn't include long-term care and doesn't necessarily pay for it. The government may not have the financial means to look after all of us as we age. In the third chapter of *Neglected No More*, Picard outlines the cost of care in Ontario. I can tell you that as most seniors age and hopefully have very little if any mortgage debt, the majority are certainly putting out a lot less than $2,700 per month for their accommodations, which seems to be an average amount of money for a basic assisted living suite in many provinces, and that does not include any type of "care." I know of clients who spend up to $15,000 per month on living arrangements depending on the facility and type of care required. Keep in mind that as of 2023, the Canada Pension Plan MAXIMUM benefit is $1,306.57 with an Old Age Security supplement of $687.56, which is less than $2000 per month of income. If my own father did not have a pension, he certainly would not be able to afford his $2,700 plus assisted living rent and expenses. He would then need to rely on family financial support or have a very limited choice of housing with government, income tested subsidization.

Today, low-income seniors can apply for subsidies, but those subsidies only cover the basic accommodation, which can sometimes mean living in a room with three other adults. It's impossible to know what future subsidies may or may not look like, or if they will even exist at all. We're at a critical point in time where if we don't plan individually, there's going to be a collective waiting list for long-term care beds clogging up hospital systems and thus limiting access to acute care facilities. Also, the quality of the care, which has been questioned in the pandemic aftermath, is uncertain, as the country has seen unprecedented losses of *all* frontline workers in *every* industry, including healthcare. So, when seniors go from living independently in their own, *paid-for home*, and now become frail and require institutionalization, this is a very costly endeavour that some seniors have not adequately prepared for. As mentioned above, some luxury seniors' residences could cost as much as $15,000 per month depending on services available and care requirements. So, it behooves us to consider these costs while we are still young enough to afford to proactively plan. The type of existence and lifestyle we desire will factor into how we plan for our final twenty to thirty years of life.

The cost and chances of living in an institution dramatically increases in our last ten to fifteen years of life, and it makes sense financially and for our collective well-being, to try and prevent frailty and thus institutionalization, if it is at all possible.

The strategy of preventing institutionalization (long-term care placement) is possible. It includes some of the following proactive approaches:

Prevention of disease and hospitalization by:

a. getting immunized (strategies used since 1796 for small pox)	a. periodic hearing assessments (decreases risk of cognitive decline)
b. tobacco and alcohol cessation programs	c. regular dental care (bad teeth are bad for inflammation and the heart)
d. regular exercise (often underrated as a therapeutic entity)	e. knowing and reviewing your risk factors for cardiovascular disease
f. adequate nutritional goals (being realistic about ideal weight and long-term benefits)	g. managing/reducing known manageable cardiovascular risks
h. monitoring blood pressures (available through pharmacies and self purchased)	i. prevention of frailty (why I wrote this book)
j. monitoring blood sugars (available only with lab work from clinician or insurance lab work or glucometer of a family member)	k. prevention of falls (hopefully this will also be a noted result from interventions in this book)
l. keep adequately hydrated (keeping in mind your age, the environment, activity levels, weight and medical conditions like congestive heart failure, kidney or liver dysfunction)	m. keeping crucial networks and social interactions intact as we get older and possibly, creating new intergenerational connections
n. getting appropriate sleep for age and activity levels, preferably without any additional medications	o. creating your own "reason for being" or Ikagai as the Japanese call this concept
p. regular vision assessments (especially important for diabetes and hypertension to look for occult end organ damage)	q. reducing hospitalization and the detrimental adverse effects of hospital acquired deconditioning and other hazards of hospitalization/immobility (pneumonia, blood clots, medication adverse events, hospital acquired delirium/pathogens/diseases etc)

So, staying in one's own home (aging in place) is the goal for many seniors. That being said, I know in my own family, moving to an assisted living residence has been nothing but a blessing for my father, as the social interactions and activities could not be offered if he remained in his own home alone. Health care teams often see when some help in the home is required, but if family resources are limited or absent, it results in a deterioration in overall condition of the senior client. While home care services are available in each province, the reliability of the service and its limitations have been called into question, especially with the pandemic and the post pandemic reduction in human resources. There are also funding limitations to home care services provincially that also limit access to this needed service. If we, as seniors, want to stay in our own home until the end, how can we do this without enough home care support for our aging population from the local health authorities as funded by provincial and federal governments? This may be an additional expense that proactively, the senior needs to research and plan for.

Across this country, and in many other countries, there are limited government funded resources for caring for the frail seniors in the community. Once the client exhausts the daily maximum amount of care, then placement into long-term care is suggested, as there is more funding allocated to long-term care than home care services. This, however, is not what most elders want.

While I am *not* a financial expert, I have taken additional training in insurance and investing. I successfully completed the LLQP exam[5] in 2015. This financial-services basic requirement exam has given me great insight into what I would've done differently if I'd had all this information at a much younger age. The financial circumstances and potential strategies that will be discussed in this book come from my experience as a veteran health care provider dealing with complicated health and financial circumstances. Rest assured, all financial details in this book have been reviewed with a certified financial planner. These suggestions are simply guidelines to open the communications for further dialogue with a team of professionals to help you plan for care as individuals age.

---

5   Life License Qualification Program

I strongly believe that one's financial care should parallel their health care.

If we are fortunate, we'll have a primary care provider who will consult specialists as needed and refer to our specialty trained allied health professionals for physiotherapy, nutritional and dietary assessment, occupational therapy, mental health assessment, and other services if required.

In financial care, your certified financial planner (CFP) acts like your primary care provider. The CFP would be as comprehensive as your family doctor or nurse practitioner in getting to know your financial health/status. Your CFP will then ask you to liaise with your accountant, lawyer, financial institution, or other tax or estate specialists, just like your primary care provider will refer to specialists and other professionals. There are many advantages to working with a certified financial planner[6] as we go through life. Those details are beyond the scope of this book, but I would ask you to verify this with your own CFP and ask for details about the evidence and benefits of working with this very important class of professionals.

The number of team members involved in providing top notch health and financial care to a senior can be overwhelming. Some seniors have this all under control because they've been slowly doing these tasks as circumstances change in their lives. I would say that by the time we're fifty years old, these tasks should be initiated if not completed, especially having a will and power of attorney (POA) identified. We have no way of knowing how long we're on this earth for, but often the ride stops abruptly. I've seen it every workday for the last four decades, and unfortunately, advanced age isn't necessarily a predictor of tragic outcomes. Let's think ahead and be prepared for that day so that our loved ones have one less task on their plate and can grieve their loss without additional stressors.

On the next page, I've included a diagram showing the interactions between your business team members and have paralleled this with your health-care team members. If this appears overwhelming, remember that you may not need all those services just yet. You can slowly seek

---

6   fpcanada.ca.

out those business professionals that you want as part of your team. It doesn't have to be done all at once, unless you leave it until your last few months of living. Be proactive and start your planning now.

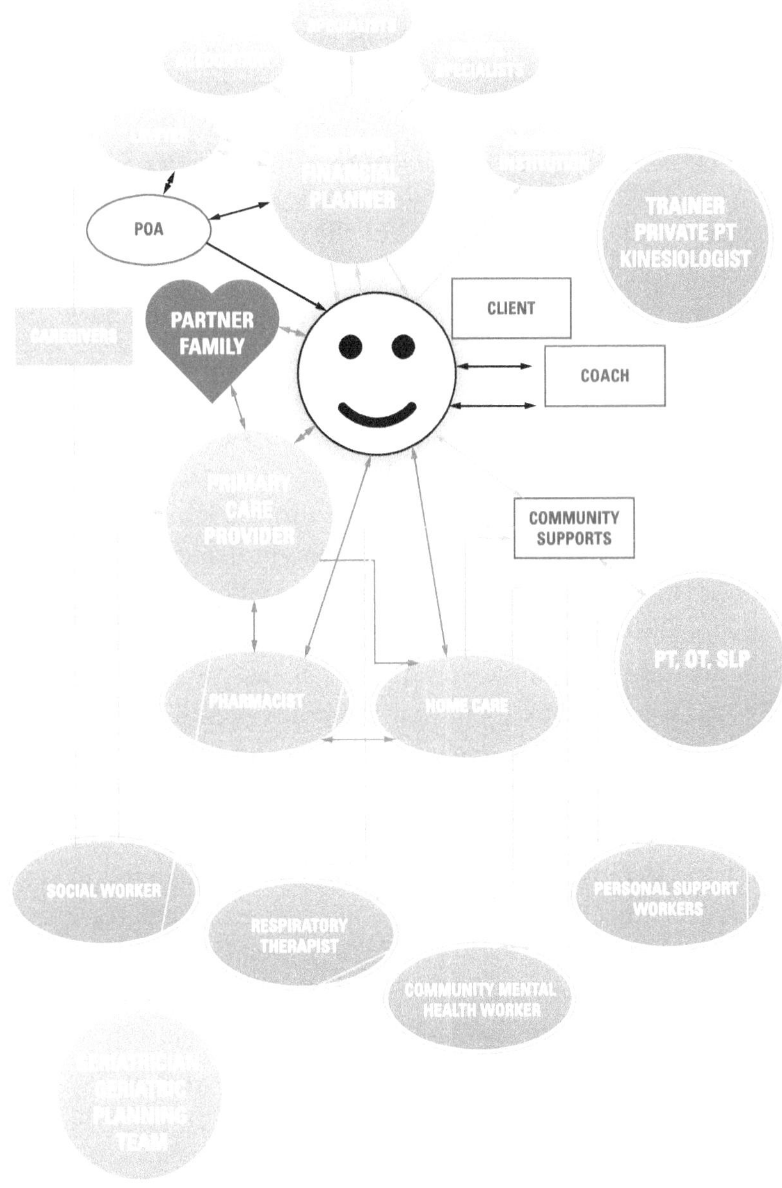

Please take the time to review the diagram and use it as a guide to keep track of who you have on your team. Remember that your primary care provider, physician, or nurse practitioner will be the "quarterback" of your health-care team. Specialists are considered "offensive coordinators" (if you follow football) and give advice and an overall game plan that may need to be adjusted by your quarterback.

While you may think that your financial planner is "there to make you rich," your financial planner is your quarterback for your financial health, wealth, estate, and tax planning issues that arise. The lawyer, accountant, other tax, and estate specialists are the "offensive coordinators" on the financial side of the game of life.

Why should you listen to me? I have been a lifetime caregiver. I've worked in healthcare for about forty years, starting in the early 1980s as a nurse in Manitoba, and I've continued to work in healthcare over the last twenty-five years as an internal medicine specialist, both in Manitoba and British Columbia. I've worked in nursing homes where I was responsible for medication administration for *an unsafe* number of patients in the early years! I've provided care in community settings, acute care centres, urban centres, rural and remote centres, and assisted living and long-term care centres. I've always been aware that the quality of care provided in care homes across Canada varies widely and has been under-funded for at least the last fifty years. While this is not a book about how to improve funding or care at the institutional level, I am actively encouraging advocacy at all levels of society for these improvements, starting today!

I will speak of the things that individuals and families can do to prevent this decline into frailty. This book is targeted at adults who are near mid life. But anyone with an interest in eldercare in the population should read this book. This is a period when there are still lots of planning options available for the future and the last thirty to forty years of life. It will also assist these mid-life adults in caring for their elderly loved ones today, who perhaps only have ten to fifteen years of life left. I feel that we must educate, encourage, and enable all adults to advocate about the concepts of *appropriate elder care.* Community members in their fifties and older can start working toward a strategy to improve eldercare. By starting today, the quality of this care will hopefully, incrementally improve every year going forward. My age, at the time of writing this book, is sixty years old. I can say with certainty, that almost all the suggestions in this book have been incorporated into my own personal life. As a clinician, there are very few presentations that one works on, that doesn't change the practice of the individual care provider. This is the ongoing educational component of health care providers. Our learning and teaching will never truly be done! As I reflect on the preparation done to prepare for this book, I could absolutely see the benefit of incorporating these suggestions into my own life. I will reflect upon my own journey on this road to frailty prevention in Chapter 17.

I hope to illustrate through the clinical scenarios the anticipated *best-case* outcomes of interventions that will be successful in improving our health as we age. As an adult medicine specialist, I've been active in providing exercise prescriptions to clients who undertake stress testing for fitness assessment, cardiovascular disease, diabetes, and obesity. During my research for this book, I've found that cardiac exercise alone won't prevent frailty. There are many other domains of interventions that society needs to incorporate for frailty prevention. Some of these include strength or resistance training, balance exercises, brain exercises, home assessments (looking at how one functions safely in the home), appropriate medication prescribing as individuals age, and comprehensive geriatric assessments in many subgroups of individuals. Social prescribing is a new term that assists in to enhancing everyone's social connectedness. We all need to feel that we "belong" to something or some group. We are social creatures by nature. The pandemic exposed just how vulnerable single seniors have been, and we (the community) need to collectively ensure that isolation from family and friends is a concept of the past. I will address social issues as part of each scenario discussion.

Finally, there are distinct advocacy plans that the taxpayers and voters need to push as political agenda items so that we can collectively improve the status of overall health care in our population in our current state but also as we all age.

I am open to other ideas readers may see as appropriate in order to facilitate change and improve quality of lives. My goal is to start a wave of inspiration and open dialogue, so that communities and societies engage in conversations that will ultimately improve elder care. Time is of the essence – every day, more of us will need care unless we do something different and something soon!

So why don't we all get started?

CHAPTER 1:
FRAILTY DEFINITIONS AND DETAILS

The aim is to postpone frailty, postpone degenerative disease, debilitation and so on and thereby shortening the period at the end of life, which is passed into decrepit or disabled state, while extending life as a whole.
—Aubrey de Grey[7] (English author, biomedical gerontologist, and author on aging)

What is frailty and how is it assessed?

It's been recognized in North American and European medical literature that frailty has been described with varying prevalence in populations greater than sixty-five years of age. A recent Statistics Canada report shows that twenty-two percent of the community dwelling population over sixty-five is identified as frail.[8] Women have more illnesses and frailty; however, men who are frail have a higher mortality rate.[9] In the end, more women outlive men and will eventually require long-term care. The breakdown of British Columbia's long term care summary is available from the Office of the Seniors Advocate.

For the health care practitioners reviewing this subject, frailty results from an aging related syndrome of decline in physiological processes. This results in an older individual becoming vulnerable to negative health outcomes. Frail older patients present with an obvious degree of generalized weakness, fatigue, medical complexity, and reduced tolerance to medications and medical/surgical procedures. Frailty is associated with a higher mortality rate in many studies published in European and North American medical journals. It's considered to be the syndrome that predisposes individuals to cognitive decline,

---

7   De Grey, Aubrey "Life Extension Strategies Beyond Calorie Restriction" *Nutrition Reviews*, 2009.

8   https://www150.statcan.gc.ca/n1/pub/82-003-x/2021004/article/00002-eng.htm

9   Ibid.

delirium, disability, falls, fractures, hospitalization, incontinence, institutionalization, poor surgical outcomes, and sadly, mortality.

While I think everyone has a mental picture of a frail older adult, frailty is actually *not a normal part of aging*. There are two ways to look at frailty. One is the subjective and physical signs of frailty, which would be somebody who has fatigue, weight loss, low activity levels, and slow gait. The second is a functional description of frailty is a combination of notable medical conditions and complexities, and the inability to do certain functional tasks in everyday existence. In the medical literature, this is termed, deficit accumulation frailty, or index frailty.

The calculations for frailty can be done by health care teams and there are many validated scoring systems that can reproducibly identify the most frail, vulnerable older adults. But these clinical and functional deficits come from the interactions of a multitude of different factors that could include medical, educational, environmental, and psychological issues. These can be longstanding entities that may or may not be amenable to treatment. The end result is reduced functional status—which **possibly** can be improved. It is the potential for improvement in frailty and functional status, which is the ultimate goal of this book. Impaired physiological reserve, which is the ability to successfully respond to medical, surgical, and other stressors, is more of a complex issue and may not always be improved due to the complex biochemical processes (at the cellular level) that accompany long standing diseases and aging. But these physiologic processes, if allowed to decline and without activity and other interventions, would ultimately lead to the progression of this vulnerable state and the negative consequences or outcomes that are now well known to be associated with frailty.

Frailty exists on a spectrum. Robust is what I would like to achieve, but I am not so certain that running a marathon at the age of ninety is my personal goal! The transition from robust to prefrail, frail, failure to thrive/pre terminal will occur at a *reduced rate of decline*, if we can limit those frailty features that are modifiable.

When clients are considered frail, the job of the individuals, families, and primary care providers is to rule out any curable or

treatable conditions, to improve quality of life and possibly longevity. This approach requires the team of the client, family members, allied health care providers, and primary care provider to know the client's baseline functional status and determine if any deterioration is occurring in a rapid or sustained manner. In my role as an adult medicine specialist, I think we can improve a senior's quality of life, if the team uncovers undiagnosed depression, rheumatologic disease (such as polymyalgia rheumatica), cardiovascular diseases (such as congestive heart failure), or underlying malignancy. While we might not change the outcome of the malignancy, getting an early diagnosis is critical to review possible treatment options before the client's general decline. Many options for chemotherapy depend on the individual's performance status at the time of diagnosis.[10] It also allows clients to focus on the quality of life (bucket list plans, etc.) if they know that their timeframe is going to be markedly less than what they thought they had.

While depression is treatable, there's still a lack of social acceptance of mental illness in our population and a greater lack of access to mental health professionals. Some famous sports figures are just starting to reach out to the public and normalize the high prevalence of mental health disorders in society, but I find that older clients are somewhat reserved in accepting that they might have depression. Health-care providers have been, historically, suboptimal champions for looking after their own or their colleagues own physical and mental health needs. As access to health care affects all community members, access to mental health services is no different and likely becoming more important given the post pandemic mental health effects that the studies are now showing. The two years of our global pandemic with COVID-19 has certainly brought to light the increase in mental health deterioration in all persons, in all age groups, and in all professions in the community. There has been an increase in social isolation, weight gain, alcohol use, and the need for mental health

---

10 "ECOG Performance Status Scale," ECOG-ACRIN, Cancer Research Group, accessed August 22, 2022, https://ecog-acrin.org/resources/ecog-performance-status/#:~:text=The%20ECOG%20Performance%20Status%20Scale,%2C%20working%2C%20etc.).

services. While I will briefly discuss some depression assessments that individuals can do on their own, I would encourage anyone who is depressed or suicidal to seek out their local community mental health worker or physician, or go to the nearest emergency room if your suicidal thoughts are active. The **Canada Suicide Prevention Service number** is **1-833–456–4566**.

An individual uses the most health care resources in their existence during the final year of life. But people don't know if this is the final curtain call when they present to the hospital with their heart attack, exacerbation of COPD, pneumonia, fall, or CHF exacerbation. One *never* knows when the last few months of life are going to be. Sometimes astute individuals will know that their time is limited to days or weeks, but most patients feel that they'll survive and bounce back. My own mother, full of cancer, heart failure, and blood clots, never acknowledged that she wasn't going to go back home. It was a particularly traumatic end for my mom, because it was only when numerous nurses and physicians failed to secure intravenous access, after trying to get that invasive access on numerous parts of her body, that she herself, finally conceded that she was done with these painful procedures. Only then, did she agree to go to a palliative care bed. She fell asleep with her soul mate of sixty-two years present, and she died peacefully ten hours after she went into palliative care. While many frail clients will get out of hospital and go back home, they often go home in worse shape due to hospital-acquired deconditioning and new medications being prescribed. Some of these frail folks continue to bounce back … until they don't. The mortality rate in Canada and other countries increases with age but also with increasing levels of frailty.[11]

There isn't a day that goes by that I don't read a news article about identifying frailty.[12] In hospital settings, identification of frailty without

---

11 "Association of Frailty and Pre-frailty with Increased Risk of Mortality among Older Canadians," April 21, 2021, https://www150.statcan.gc.ca/n1/pub/82-003-x/2021004/article/00002-eng.pdf.

12 "Faster Diagnosis of Frailty in Seniors Aging at Home Is Key to Helping Them Stay Independent," The Conversation, April 7, 2022, https://theconversation.com/faster-diagnosis-of-frailty-in-seniors-aging-at-home-is-key-to-helping-them-stay-independent-177246.

an intensive plan to decrease frailty has proven futile. As a clinician, I feel that health care providers need to focus on:

- *identifying* frailty,
- *investigating* for treatable conditions,
- *improving* therapies for known conditions,
- *initiating interventions* that will start benefiting these folks, and then
- evaluating/documenting *improvements* in frailty scores, outcomes, and quality of life and other metrics.

I call this Dr. Karen's *5-I plan.*

There are more than sixty frailty assessment tools currently available, but there is no one current gold standard. I find an easy tool to use is the FRAIL score,[13] which is a score between 0–5.

#1 F	Have you felt FATIGUED most or all of the time over the last month?	Yes = 1	No = 0	SCORE
#2 R	RESISTANCE. Do you have any difficulty climbing a flight of stairs?	Yes = 1	No = 0	
#3 A	ACTIVITY/AMBULATION. Do you have difficulty walking one block?	Yes = 1	No = 0	
#4 I	How many of the following ILLNESSES do you have? Hypertension, diabetes, cancer, chronic lung disease, heart disease, congestive heart failure, heart attack, angina, asthma, arthritis, stroke, kidney disease	5+ = 1	less than 5 = 0	
#5 L	Have you LOST greater than five percent of your body weight in the last year?	Yes = 1	No = 0	

A score of 0 would indicate that the individual is robust. A score of 1–2 would indicate some pre-frailty status. And a score of 3–5 would suggest that these individuals have been screened as frail, with 5 being the most severe frail category. Anything other than robust needs interventions to be initiated now! In the hospital setting, there is an entire TEAM dedicated to this goal of identifying frailty and getting some interventions lined up for the hospital stay and for a

---

13 J.E. Morley and T.K. Malstrom, "A Simple Frailty Questionnaire (FRAIL) Predicts Outcomes in Middle Aged African Americans," National Library of Medicine, July 25, 2015, https://www.ncbi.nlm.nih.gov/pmc/articles/PMC4515112/.

short time frame post discharge. This of course, depends on where the senior lives and outpatient accessibility to these services.

But what about those individuals that do not have access to care and are not ill enough to require hospitalization? What can individuals, family members, concerned friends do outside of the institutional setting to identify the frail folks in their world?

From my perspective, using a basic scoring system is reasonable.

Do your own FRAIL score or that of the elderly person in your life. Tally up the points. If you're robust, fantastic! Keep doing what you're doing. If you're pre-frail, we need to get to work! If you're frail, we need to come up with a plan to try and get you back to the pre-frail category if possible, and ideally back to robust!

In general, being fatigued, not being able to climb one flight of stairs, not being able to walk one block, losing a significant amount of weight, *unintentionally*, and having numerous comorbid conditions are what we need to know to define frailty outside of being in care.

How do we improve this score to the point so that somebody is no longer considered frail? This is the focus on the following chapters of the book to give individuals and care givers a basic recipe as a starting point, for addressing frailty. As the book evolves, readers will see how to advance the recipe in order to achieve a "less frail" status.

With the frailty scoring system I use, the most concerning symptom for an adult of any age is unintentional weight loss. As a specialist, I believe that the first thing care givers should do is consider the list of the causes for unintentional weight loss or malnutrition in older adults. We need to review medications, assess for illnesses such as underlying malignancy or systemic diseases, depression with or without paranoia, alcoholism (sometimes difficult to ascertain without collateral history from friends or family), swallowing issues, oral cavity issues such as tongue lesions, canker sores, poor fitting dentures, lack of money for food, the presence of wandering (burning excess calories), dementia or forgetting the need or importance of eating, hyperthyroidism, malabsorption, functional act of eating issues (tremor, stroke, weakness), restrictive diets and shopping or food preparation problems.

If you use an Internet search engine to read about frailty, you will often find calculators for clinicians to grade or calculate frailty. These are not necessarily helpful to family members or seniors themselves. Sometimes, readers will find a term called Frailty Index.[14] This is a scoring system used in geriatrics research and was even used as a Statistics Canada survey in 2013/2014 when the government sent out a frailty scoring system consisting of thirty questions. This study was published in April 2021, and a copy is available by doing a literature search. It is essentially a math value calculated by identifying the number of deficits an individual has divided by the number of deficits considered. For the purpose of general education of frailty in this book, these scoring systems are beyond the scope of what individuals and family members need to know about their unique family situation. However, as a guideline for general knowledge, the FRAILTY INDEX scoring system identified clients as not frail (<0.21), robust (0–0.10), pre-frail (0.11–0.21), frail (>0.21), moderately frail (0.22–0.44), and most frail (>0.45). The Statistics Canada report also correlated mortality rates with those subclasses of frailty versus not frail.

For clinicians, there are many other screening tools used in frailty assessments that may include gait speed testing, grip strength testing, and many other questionnaires that are available from the Comprehensive Geriatric Assessment (CGA) toolkit which is also available on the Internet.

In the clinical setting, I use some of the tests from the CGA toolkit that look at walking speed, general mobility, and overall strength. This is also coupled with a neuromuscular exam to determine if any motor, sensory or neurologic impairments are present.

I love the ease of testing and the simple directions that are available on the GCAtoolkit.com website. I encourage all readers to review this website if further information is required.

I like to use the scoring systems for educating individuals about what slow movements can mean in real world risk terms. I also like

---

14 "Association of Frailty and Pre-frailty with Increased Risk of Mortality among Older Canadians," April 21, 2021, https://www150.statcan.gc.ca/n1/pub/82-003-x/2021004/article/00002-eng.pdf.

the sarcopenia screening questionnaire as it illustrates to the senior how concerning repeated falls can be to the individual. Again, these systems are part of a more comprehensive geriatric assessment. However, given the limitations of access to geriatricians, I believe that self assessment (senior or family member) and proactively seeking out a safer strategy to improve these objective assessments, could go far in preventing the frailty progression and complications like falls.

Scoring for a gait speed test (over 4 metres) includes some of the following factors:

1. Less than 10 seconds = normal;
   a. caveat = Greater than 10 seconds = predictive of near falls in older adults with hip osteoarthritis
2. 10–20 seconds = good mobility. Can go out alone. Mobile without a gait aid.
   a. Caveat = Greater than 14 seconds = associated with high fall risk in community dwelling for frail older adults.
3. 10–30 seconds = impaired mobility. Likely needs a gait aid (cane, walker or other)
   a. Caveat = Greater than 24 seconds = predictive of falls within six months after a hip fracture.
4. Greater than 30 seconds = severely impaired mobility. Cannot go outside alone. Requires a gait aid.
   a. Caveat= Greater than 30 seconds = predictive of requiring an assistive device for ambulation and being dependent in activities of daily living

Muscle Strength and Fall Assessment

	Question	Scoring	Score
STRENGTH	How much difficulty do you have in lifting and carrying ten pounds?	None = 0 Some = 1 A lot or unable to = 2	
ASSISTANCE NEEDED	How much difficulty do you have walking across a room?	None = 0 Some = 1 A lot, uses aids, or unable = 2	
CHAIR MOBILITY	How much difficulty do you have when transferring from a chair or bed?	None = 0 Some = 1 A lot or unable = 2	
ACTIVITY WITH STAIRS	How much difficulty do you have climbing a flight of ten stairs?	None = 0 Some = 1 A lot or unable = 2	
OVERALL FALL RISK	How many times have you fallen in the past year?	None = 0 Some (1-2) = 1 A lot or unable (3+) =2	

A score equal to or greater than 4 is predictive of profound muscle weakness, falls and poor health outcomes.

Please calculate your own score, and if your score is > 0, then some of the exercise prescriptions that are noted later in this book can be utilized to hopefully improve your overall strength. If your score is more than 4, then a referral to an outpatient physiotherapy program, after being reviewed by your primary care provider to rule out any possible neuromuscular disorders, and initiating an exercise program when medically cleared would be prudent. If you are already in the 7–8 zone, preservation of your overall strength, if not improving it, should be anticipated. However, if you're bedridden and falling, or have a score of 9 or 10, you will need a modified approach because of your underlying limitations, and this will be discussed later in the book.

What is sarcopenia?

This is a term used to describe age-related loss in skeletal muscle.[15] While there is a known age-related reduction in muscle as a direct

---

15 W.J. Evans, "What Is Sarcopenia?" National Library of Medicine, November 1995, https://pubmed.ncbi.nlm.nih.gov/7493218/.

cause of the decrease in muscle strength, muscle mass (not function) is thought to be the major determinant of decreases in strength as we age. With advancing age and the extremely low activity level seen in the very old, muscle strength is a critical component of walking ability. The main determinant of energy expenditure is fat-free mass, which declines by about fifteen percent between the third and eighth decade of life, contributing to the lower basal metabolic rate in the elderly. Preservation of muscle mass and preventing the development of sarcopenia, can help prevent the known decrease in metabolic rate. There are known consequences like that fact that skeletal muscle and its age-related decline may contribute to such age-associated changes such as reduced bone density (osteoporosis), decreased insulin sensitivity, and general reduction in overall cardiovascular (aerobic) capacity. Hopefully some interventions to improve or delay muscle deterioration will be helpful in maintaining fitness, which would ideally result in less frailty, falls, fractures, hospitalization, institutionalization, and death. These are the concepts that I wish to promote to hopefully improve the expectations of an aging population and to provide an implementation guide for activity plans, so that functional improvement can occur en masse.

Not being able to walk quickly is another single objective test of frailty and should be used with other data. Ideally, this test is done by a healthcare professional, but family members who understand the test may assess the individual to see how well they're doing. Walking speed is important for adults who use walking as their primary means of transportation. Safely getting through the pedestrian crosswalk in time will help reduce further risk when ambulating alone. The test can be performed with any patient able to walk four metres. The patient is to walk at their normal pace using their normal assistive device as per their usual walking routine. The individual being tested is to be timed walking through a four-metre walking zone with a short distance marked out for acceleration and deceleration. The time walking in the middle four meters is timed.

Gait speed is total distance/time, and a gait speed of 0.8 m/s or less is considered abnormal and will require further assessment with clinicians or outpatient community therapy services.

One of the many definitions of frailty includes decreased physical activity, as identified kilocalories spent per week. For men, this is expending less than 380 kcal per week, and for women, it's less than 270 kcal per week. Other objective data could include a slow walking speed greater than six to seven seconds to walk fifteen feet, and assessing grip strength (there are age-appropriate norms identified for grip strength using a dynamometer available online if readers are interested).

In this next table, I have tabulated some basic low-level activities to help one estimate energy utilization per week depending on the activity. More activities are listed on various websites if other information is required.

Activity	Kcal used per 30 minutes	Comments
Walking 2.5 mph	100	Easiest to determine on treadmill
Walking 3 mph	142	Easiest to determine on treadmill
Walking 3.7	191	Easiest to determine on treadmill
Calisthenics light/moderate	167	Uptake range of calories expended depending on the aggressiveness of the workload
Raking lawn	208	Sometimes an enjoyable task given the calories used
Gardening	167	This is also a mental health activity for the author
Vacuuming	160	This is a necessary evil
Wash Car	142	This is when the author's husband wants to hide from other chores
Cleaning	100	Another necessary evil, sometimes therapeutic
Sex, foreplay	21	Not much calories burned, but contributes to quality of life
Sex	208	Many partners would suggest that every couple needs to do more of this activity

While a lot of these mobility assessments help with overall physical frailty assessments, it's also a marker of driver safety if the elderly person is still driving a motor vehicle. In many jurisdictions, there are distinct medical assessments required to be completed by the primary care provider after a certain age. Gait mobility alone shouldn't be the only indication for restricting driving. Neck and shoulder mobility, overall energy level, fatiguability and drowsiness, how an individual responds reflexively to changing driving situations, understanding the road markings and road direction changes, problem solving, and being aware of location and circumstances are all critical in driving. For families and clients alike, limiting someone's driving is one of the most distressing events as an individual ages. The perception that they are being discriminated against based on age alone causes anger and agitation. However, the reality is that if you develop frailty, you shouldn't be driving. Before frailty develops, clients and families must discuss the circumstances under which the client will need to give up driving. The sooner this is discussed in a family situation, the better the client and family will be prepared to come up with alternative solutions for transportation. In the case of cognitive impairment, documentation of these conversations for the client is critical, so that there is a reference of when this was discussed. As a physician, I am legally obligated to report when I feel someone is no longer fit to drive. It's nothing personal. It's about doing my part to keep the roads as safe as possible for all passengers and pedestrians. In my jurisdiction, there are local websites listing the standards prescribed by the government.[16]

Getting back to the frailty scoring system I use; fatigue is also another concerning symptom.

While there's no sure-fire fix for fatigue and fatigability, there is the ability to improve balance, flexibility, resistance, and endurance with weight loss, exercise, and sound nutrition. Some fatigue improves with

---

16 "Senior Drivers," Government of British Columbia, accessed August 22, 2022, https://www2.gov.bc.ca/gov/content/transportation/driving-and-cycling/roadsafetybc/medical-fitness/seniors#:~:text=To%20keep%20our%20roads%20safe%2C%20all%20drivers%20must,and%20better.%20Approximately%2098%25%20keep%20their%20driving%20privileges.

an enhanced cardiovascular fitness level and/or weight loss. But for people with chronic medical conditions, the fatigue can be the most difficult symptom to manage. There are no reliable or safe "uppers," otherwise I would be on one. The fatigue aspect is especially true with chronic liver disease but also can occur with any chronic organ disease, such as chronic kidney disease, ischemic heart disease, diabetes, and congestive heart failure. The comorbid conditions can be optimized with medications and possibly other interventions. The fatigue may also be caused by certain medications. Health-care providers should only prescribe medications where there is a *clear indication* for the benefit of quality or quantity of life, as per the client's own directions.

Enhancing socialization and working on brain activities are essential tools that we need to add to our longevity toolbox. This may also assist in treating depression that could also be manifested as fatigue. Many people are resistant to change and are anchored in their daily habits and routines. Some of us are stubborn and can't be bothered to maintain friendships and relationships. Our job as caregivers is to explore those behaviours to uncover undiagnosed depression, abuse, or other concerning issues. If any kind of abuse is suspected, please contact the Canadian Network for Prevention of Elder Abuse (CNPEA) or a similar program in your jurisdiction. The Seniors Abuse and Information Line (SAIL) is toll free at 1-866-437-1940. If you know someone who is being neglected or abused in any way, please call 911 if it's a life-threatening event, or call the SAIL line for assistance. *Please!*

In the next chapter, we'll review the history of the problem, and in subsequent chapters, we'll outline the basic principles of interventions that can delay frailty onset or improve pre-frail status to less frail. We'll discuss clinical scenarios with many age groups represented and examine potential action plans and activity prescriptions, socialization plans, advocacy options, and financial implications for each scenario.

CHAPTER SUMMARY

We have reviewed some of the frailty assessment tools and scoring systems that are usually done at the professional/geriatrician level when we have identified significant frailty concerns. But not all clients have access to geriatrician assessments. I hope that by reading this chapter, you will understand some of the factors that health-care professionals look at in assessing frailty as we age. You can then make your own assessment about how frail you or your loved one might be. Every individual knows if they can climb stairs, cross a room, or walk a block. Most of us understand how our clothes fit when we experience unexpected weight loss. Many family members recognize that their older loved ones are frail, and now they have some objective tools to start looking at the specifics and to seek out assistance from health-care or other professionals as the picture becomes clearer or circumstances arise. Finally, the safe ability to drive is impaired with frailty. Wouldn't keeping your independence with being able to drive be a key motivator for frailty prevention?

CHAPTER 2:
CURRENT HEALTH CARE LIMITATIONS AS THE POPULATION AGES

If you shift your focus from yourself to others, extend your concern to others, and cultivate the thought of caring for the well-being of others, then this will have the immediate effect of opening up your life and helping you reach out. —Dalai Lama XIV[17]

While the majority of elderly people want to stay in their own homes to the end, I know first hand how beneficial moving in with other seniors can be from the social interaction perspective. As young adults going to college or university, we were excited to leave home and venture out or co-habitate with similar aged adults. Why does moving to a retirement residence, assisted living, or long-term care home have to viewed differently and with such angst?

I want to engage you to come up with a strategy to assist any elderly person in your life to determine what is important to that elder and help them achieve their latter life goals. I feel this is URGENTLY required as many seniors do not have any access to primary health care and this is an issue that has no guaranteed short-term resolution. I know, it seems like you might be meddling, "shouldn't I be minding my own business?" One of the simplest ways to assess which older person needs assistance is by actively listening to them when you say, "I notice that your lawn has not been mowed for a few weeks. Is there anything that I can do to help?" You may uncover a lot of care issues by opening a conversation and listening to what is going poorly in that person's life. You do not have to commit to anything, but you could discuss the situation with this person's family members, if you are given the permission to do so. Often, families who are not nearby have very little idea about how the elder is actually doing.

---

17 The Dalai Lama XIV, 1998; "The Art of Happiness."

Historically, women have outnumbered men in care homes due to their higher average lifespan. However, societal, and cultural influences, combined with a lack of exercise and motivation in the advanced age groups, tends to result in women having a higher prevalence of frailty. While getting older doesn't imply that we will automatically become frail, certain conditions exist that promote frailty. In the last chapter we explored a few of the scoring systems that you can use to identify frailty in yourself, your own family members, and the population. The focus on the rest of the book is how we, as a community, rise to the challenge of promoting a more robust existence as we age.

While I like the simplicity of the FRAIL score, there are many other scoring systems that I alluded to in the last chapter. In 2013/2014, the Government of Canada (Statistics Canada) used the frailty index scoring system.[18] In April 2021, the report from that data estimated that the prevalence of frailty was twenty-two percent in those aged sixty-five years old and older. Sadly, as people become frailer, the report also illustrated that mortality rate increases with increasing degrees of frailty. As we have seen over the last ten years, this has led to a large burden of morbidity and mortality in our healthcare system. This is evidenced by the degree of overcapacity in almost all acute care hospitals and an increasing burden of ALC patients, which are folks waiting for an alternate level of care bed. This system has been fragile for years, but the global pandemic made obvious the shortcomings in healthcare systems across the country. In Canada, and in my province of British Columbia, we have a primary care crisis. The number of critical primary care providers that provide longitudinal care to their clients has been slowly dwindling for years. This is a complex problem present in every community and the majority of our country. While the government is trying to activate short-term fixes as soon as possible, in the long term, there needs to be a different model of care and increased training of not only primary care providers, but also increased training and numbers of all members of the health-care team. When training is completed, there needs to be reasonable working conditions. For physicians, it would include clinic expenses, wages,

18 https://www150.statcan.gc.ca/n1/pub/82-003-x/2021004/article/00002-eng.htm

quality of life, and work-life balance. These are just a few of the factors required to sustain a long-term service, that isn't disrupted every few months or years due to lack of human resources. Clinics need concrete contingency plans for patients when care providers go on vacations, sabbaticals, parental leaves, sick leaves, general leaves of absences, and retirement. Having these plans in place may also assist with hopefully, delaying the onset of burnout, which today, is *highly* prevalent in all health-care providers. In my own experience, this type of care exists in community health centres (CHCs). I believe these types of care models will improve the access and quality of care to all Canadians.

The lack of primary health care means that individuals have no primary care provider, which could be a general or family practice physician, a physician assistant, or nurse practitioner. In the United States, there is at least sixty years of experience using physician assistants and it is estimated that thirty-five percent of primary care in the USA is provided by Board Certified Internal Medicine Specialists.

There are so many people who have no idea that they have undiagnosed diseases such as hypertension. This results in individuals developing end organ damage from common diseases, where an early diagnosis and treatment, could prevent or decrease the chance of long-term complications and excessive health care utilization. Once complications occur and are the presenting symptoms of a long-standing treatable disorder, this results in many years of burden to the health care system. So many community members haven't had any health care for years! This is such a sad state of affairs as early treatment of diseases such as diabetes, hypertension, obesity, and sleep apnea could prevent a great deal of future health care utilization and costs.

For those individuals that are fortunate enough to have a walk-in clinic to prescribe medications for chronic illnesses, it is the *longitudinal*, primary health care provider that knows the individual and can troubleshoot complications or adverse effects related to changing medical conditions, changing physiological processes, and aging metabolism. I will address the importance of dedicated medication reviews later in this book. It is my experience as a specialist, that these med reviews are done currently in exceptional circumstances and not as often as should be done as clients age, develop a plethora of new diagnoses and known declining physiologic processes and altered or diminished medication metabolism. While these medications reviews can be done by several members of the care giving team, it is often the primary care provider (and sometimes the client) that have ALL the details regarding the indications for the meds, what subspecialist caregiver prescribed or made the suggestion of the medication, knows the current status of liver and kidney functions which would be key to changing meds and or doses. The community pharmacist could also perform the task if all those pieces of information as described in the prior sentence, were known by the pharmacist. Often, without ALL the necessary pieces of information, medication reviews can be as detrimental to the client as no review at all. As a specialist, I believe for every prescribed medication an individual is taking, there has been CLEAR communications regarding the indication for its use and a timeframe for when it is going to be reviewed. Reviewing the necessity of each drug as we get older is important, as many drug categories don't have advanced age participants as part of the clinical trials. In addition, there is often reduced efficiency in drug metabolic pathways in chronic conditions and in the process of aging. New studies have also changed the indications of some prescribed medications. There are increasing amounts of medication interactions that also can be hazardous to older clients with certain conditions.

Due to these complications with medication prescribing in our current healthcare environment, I would ask that ALL individuals who are on any medications keep their own personal, up-to-date record of medications, medication changes, supplements, herbal medications, and samples given to the client from another provider. I would also advocate for education, by the prescriber or pharmacist, so the client can adequately record the indications for those medications. The client should also be instructed about known or documented drug intolerances, adverse events, medication changes, and additions or deletions. Also, individuals should document the name of the practitioner that made/suggested those changes and why those changes were made or suggested. Ideally, this would be something that a readily accessible electronic, up to date pharmacy profile could also do, if this information was readily available and lab work or other details could be added to such a document. At this point in time, a universal health record system is not available in many provinces, but is available in some.

We have great access to the list of drugs prescribed and filled in our provincial pharmanet system, but many people have extra meds, older prescriptions, and supplements that aren't accounted for. Sometimes patients who live near the borders of a province will have medications from outside of their province that may not be trackable. This makes accurate medication reconciliation from home, to hospital admission, hospital course, discharge medications and follow up with primary care a very difficult task to get this correct. This is often the reason medications are not continued as suggested post discharge or clients are readmitted due to medication changes or errors.

If clients live in a province with the lack of primary health care and an easily accessible inclusive provincial electronic medical record, I am also suggesting that clients carefully track medical conditions, appointments, diagnostic testing, test results, specialist appointments and all aspects of their own health care until such systems are in place and functioning well for all members of the health care team. The client needs to be the team member with ALL the details of his/her/their medical and surgical histories.

Health care is complex, and in my province, there is not currently *one* electronic medical record that can accessed by *every* clinic or hospital EMR system, although progress is being made on that plan. Clients are encouraged to stay on top of their own health issues because one never knows if their primary care provider will be working next week, next month, next year, or ever again.

I have primarily worked as an in-hospital specialist physician. Hospitalization for a new or chronic issue is often the first-time medications are prescribed. Medications are often started in hospital on older patients in a rapid manner, which often results in outpatient side effects and noncompliance of treatment. This will often lead to hospital readmission. All too frequently, there is not enough timely access for follow-up care in the community (seen in seven to ten days in their clinic post hospital discharge). There is a North American suggestion that all clients recently discharged from hospital should be reviewed in the community within seven days of hospital discharge. Readmission to hospital increases with complex medication regimens, or with the lack of medication reconciliation from home medications to hospital medications and finally medications required upon discharge and for the foreseeable future. Some of this is due to the fact that physicians don't always denote the reason why we are discharging the patient on certain drugs. The pharmacist can't access medical records, and it may take days and sometimes weeks for the discharge summary to go to the primary care provider, if the patient actually has a primary care provider. Many seniors also feel that there are vitamin and herbal supplements they have been on for years that shouldn't be discontinued. Unfortunately, this increases the risk of polypharmacy, which is detrimental to individuals as they age. A careful medication review, on a regular basis (every six to twelve months), with educational components about the rationale for use of each medication or supplement, can be beneficial to the individual, if this service can be provided and sustained.

In addition to medication issues identified above, some seniors are admitted to hospital and never return to their pre-illness functional status. This functional decline, further delays a timely discharge home as the hospital-associated deconditioning that occurs, requires additional hospital days in order to functionally improve the client to a point, where a safe discharge is possible. In Canada, there are twenty-nine long-term care beds per one thousand population age sixty-five and older. This adds up to 2,076 long-term care homes and 198,220 (2016 data) long-term care beds. Forecasting data estimates that Canada will require 454,000 long-term care bed by 2035, which is only thirteen years away. The average cost per bed of constructing new care homes is $320,000. The supply chain for materials has been significantly affected by both the pandemic plus the economy and the war overseas. I am not confident that we can increase the long-term care home capacity within that time frames.

Across British Columbia and the rest of Canada, every ward/department in every hospital is dramatically understaffed. Where do we get the physicians, nurse practitioners, nurses, allied health professionals, leaders, and other caregiver resources to add an additional 255,000+long-term care beds in just thirteen years?

Also, just think about the time constraints to build long-term care homes. It takes up to a year to build a single dwelling home, and several years to build long-term care facilities. We are in a great supply chain dilemma, and in British Columbia, even communities devasted by wildfires or floods have yet to start the rebuilding process. While there are some rapid construction care home projects[19] in Canada, I don't think we as seniors can expect an additional 255,000 care home beds in thirteen years. The skyrocketing costs of building supplies will also cause funded projects to be grossly over budget and then possibly further delayed. This is going to make wait lists for long-term care even longer than they are now, and will continue to clog acute care hospital beds with vulnerable elders having no place to go. *We must do whatever we can to slow this devasting process of anticipated care home requirements in the next thirteen years.* With this in mind, how can community members assist others to age in place and not be considered frail? That is what I hope this book will help us all understand and move forward.

To find local statistics about residential care facilities, I urge readers in British Columbia to seek out the Office of the Seniors Advocate, Residential Care Facilities—Quick Facts Directory 2018 Summary Statement.[20] To understand the history and complexity of long-term care crises over the last many years, I urge readers to go through Mr. Picard's book, *Neglected No More*, to further understand the historical aspects that led to the long-term care crisis in our country with the pandemic.

Throughout this book, I am using knowledge and experience from a four-decade-long health-care career with lots of "thought assets"

---

19 https://m.youtube.com/watch?v=xpw-diUGOPg

20 https://www.seniorsadvocatebc.ca/app/uploads/sites/4/2018/01/QuickFacts2018-Summary.pdf

and first-hand participation in the care of older adults. I feel that I have exceptional insight into how we can hopefully prevent the need for some of these long-term care beds in the next five to ten years. It makes sense to know how robust an individual is by identifying frailty status. It also follows that investigating for treatable conditions, initiating interventions that have been shown to prevent the development of frailty would be next in line. Then, identifying and improving the treatment of chronic conditions such as obesity, pre-diabetes, obstructive sleep apnea, diabetes, hypertension, stroke, kidney and liver disease, heart disease and heart failure, and inhibiting progression of those diseases before end-organ damage occurs makes absolute sense. Of course, as part of every quality improvement program, we must also evaluate if the interventions provided equate to improvements in functional status, overall care, hospitalization, and mortality. Finally, individualization of any therapeutic regimen is required to attain each individual's distinct goals of fitness and functionality, quality of life and other patient centric goals.

The focus of the next few chapters will be on what is required for one individual to age with a quality of life that is acceptable to that individual person. This requires two-way dialogue to provide that patient centric care. I'll focus on exercise prescriptions, pulmonary rehabilitation for those clients with COPD, resistance training exercises, and balance and brain training exercises as a general education to the general public. This book provides a basic level of education and instructions for getting the ball rolling and improving one's functional status. By including some of the rationale of why caregivers may recommend any of these interventions as one gets older, it is my desire to actively recruit every reader to become the most important participant of the health care team—the well informed and compliant client!

The case studies following these chapters will include a clinical scenario for one or more individuals, with an action plan that will include a variety of exercise prescriptions, possibly including progressive resistant training regimens, balance and brain training programs, special social prescribing, and advocacy considerations for these individual cases. Also included will be a summary of the significant financial implications to consider in each clinical scenario. Readers may find that one or two of the scenarios resonate with them or their family members. There are certainly numerous complicating factors to consider as we age, and each one of us has different issues to sort out. This book will highlight some of the more common themes that I have seen as a clinician. Hopefully, the readers will begin to think about their own situations, and plan for a non frail future, aging safely in place at home.

I will mention a variety of professionals, whose jobs are to provide education, consultation, and guidance as one ages. Please seek them out and start preparing *as soon as possible*. Review what your local jurisdiction and governments have to offer as you age. If you are not digitally savvy, engage a younger family member to assist you with your online searches. I want everyone to start advocating for changing the quality of eldercare in our communities. We need to start this process today.

CHAPTER SUMMARY

Hopefully after reading this chapter, all readers will acknowledge the extremely fragile health care system as it stands today. We are in a primary care crisis nationally. We individually must understand that each one of us needs to advocate for self care, self-monitoring, and become champions for better eldercare. We not only need to look out for ourselves and our families, but we also need to look out for those in our community, who do not have anyone locally, making sure that they are aging safely at home. Let's be aware of some of the more common medical conditions that creep into our lives as we age. Many of these conditions are silent killers. Unrecognized chronic conditions will eventually lead to an ever-increasing list of medical complications and utilization of the fragile, health care system. Having more than five of these conditions is a point in one of the categories in calculating frailty. We can only prevent complications if we know somebody has the disease, and because of the primary health-care crisis, we need to rely on our friends, families, and self advocacy to make sure that we are being looked after given the current circumstances. If this means buying a blood pressure machine because both your parents had hypertension at the same age as you currently are, then do it. Our primary care crisis is not likely to get better anytime soon, but we do want to make sure that everyone is looking out for everyone else.

There is an extremely important role for medication prescribing, review, and deprescribing as we age. Unless we're institutionalized, our primary care crisis will fall short in the suggested standard of care goals and medication reviews that I discussed in this chapter. Individuals need to have their own understanding and records of their medications and indications; they need to keep an up-to-date record of their overall health status.

CHAPTER 3:
KEY ESSENTIALS FOR OPTIMAL AGING

I believe that independent aging relies on three separate necessities in order to age safely at home. I call these the three Fs:

- Fitness and functionality
- Family
- Financial plans

First, we need *fitness and functionality* to keep us physically safe in our own homes. With that, we need realistic judgement and insight which reflect the markers of psychological/cognitive/emotional fitness and functionality. Without these essentials of physical and cognitive fitness/functionality, we will need to rely on one or both of the two other necessities for quality, aging in place. Most of the next few chapters will focus on assessing and achieving physical and cognitive fitness/functionality. Without this, it's unlikely that a senior will successfully thrive in their own home as age advances. When this is the case, we will need to rely on the other two Fs—*family* that the senior trusts and does *not* fear, and *financial* plans that are already in place, to cover the various costs of aging and to self-fund the care required for the advanced years in life.

If we don't have physical and cognitive fitness and functionality, we must rely on family to take us in when it becomes unsafe to stay at home alone. Over the past several decades, the capacity to look after a multi-generational family has declined due to the cost of living and the changing of societal norms. While most families have a minimum of two or more adult incomes, certain ethnic groups still value and cherish their elders and do an excellent job of making certain that they're cared for by the family. The Hawaiian culture is just one of the many cultures in which elders are honoured and younger generations feel privileged to look after their parents, aunts, uncles, grandparents, and other seniors in their lives. In my lifetime of working with patients and their families, I appreciate that truly "normal" family dynamics are rare and that all families are somewhere on the spectrum of dysfunctionality, some less dysfunctional than others and vice versa. An elder can't *fear* the family members looking after them. Any fears by the elder will need to be explored further to reduce any risk of elder abuse before any long-term living arrangements can be set in place or finalized.

Finally, if fitness and functionality, and willing family members to provide care are absent, then as an individual, one must have adequate *finances* to get the elder care you desire. Financial plans are discussed throughout the book, but advanced planning is required to make certain the finances are in place to provide care until death. Mobility aids, scooters, specialized chairs and beds, special medications or wound care costs are not predictable as we age, but they add up quickly and significantly. Then, there is the cost of assisted living, nursing care, and transition to long-term care. This cost of living often far exceeds what the senior is currently paying to stay alone in their own home.

Ideally, society would love to have all seniors with all of the three Fs—*fitness/functionality,* caring and compassionate *family* members, and adequate *financial* resources to pay for required care. At the very least, one of the three Fs is required for quality aging. If all three are absent, then there is a lack of options for the individual as he/she ages.

How does one encourage the first of the Fs—fitness and functionality? This is the one aspect that can be in the control of the senior, barring any devastating disease states that are irreversible.

I have found that in medicine, a paternalistic "I am the doctor, you are the patient" approach doesn't always yield success. In personal lives, large corporations, and people interacting with people as a whole, no one person can *get* another person to do something. I often tell my husband, "You can't make me do anything I don't want to do," and he knows it!

Looking back at trying to convince my own mom to exercise when she was younger, I didn't realize that her agoraphobia completely rendered my rational thoughts of exercise as a good habit useless when compared to her overwhelming anxiety about leaving her home. It donned on me when she passed away that she must have been in agony. The only safe place in the world was her own home, yet she was too ill and incapacitated to ever return home. She fought until the very end, and when she finally conceded to go into palliative care, her final hours were peaceful.

You can educate your elderly loved one to at least try to improve their fitness and functionality while their health is still reasonable. However, if you are trying to get your parent(s) to do anything, remember this, you are still the child. Your approach has to be sensitive, so that it does not appear that you or other family members are trying to control their lives. Just like when you were a teenager and they were advising a younger you, the messaging should relay the goal of safety. We need to protect our elders as they did us when we were young and naïve. It's the natural history of families that our patients almost always (but sadly, not every time) pass before the next generation. In Western society, we rarely openly discuss death and dying. We need to normalize that conversation so it's considered a realistic part of aging and not a pessimistic event. Having the ability to direct the plan of care as one ages is so important for all people.

We need to pre-emptively look at realist scenarios such as:

- Can the elderly person escape safely from a bedroom window in a fire?
- What are the tripping hazards in the home?
- Has there been a fall and what circumstances led to the fall?
- When does an elder become unsafe to drive?

I deal with these scenarios in my own family, and these are difficult conversations. But children or friends of an elderly person need to discuss these things in a non-confrontational manner. It's about getting the elderly parent/relative/friend to realize that sometimes their brains are still writing cheques that their bodies can't cash! Every individual believes that they can do the same things that they did ten years ago. However, this is what the mind believes, but the body often fails when trying to keep up.

Loss of independence is a topic that needs to be discussed early on and regularly, so that all family members are on the same page. A transition plan for loss of independence needs to be created well ahead of the loss. But be wary—some seniors will tell different family members different versions of a story. The family needs to compare notes and be transparent so that all involved are using the same messages, that the family members only want the best for the senior in question.

Before anyone embarks on a conversation with a cherished elderly loved one, please ask permission to start having conversations about functioning, frailty, and the possible repercussions of these discussions. If any of the topics are particularly sensitive, explore what is triggering these sensitivities. At times, I've been asked as a physician to discuss things like seniors driving, or if they can travel. When the family is with the client, I ask the client's permission to discuss these issues and, using a gentle approach, I go over the physical and emotional requirements of continuing to do certain tasks. There may also be some insurability or financial scenarios to explore. I also explain that physicians are obligated by law to report when driving could be unsafe, as there are medical standards in every province that limit driving; for example, if certain medical conditions exist. While it's easy for me to submit paperwork about a documented condition, it's far more difficult to tell someone they can't drive. If I believe their cognition is starting to fail, they're unable to turn their head to shoulder-check when changing lanes, their reaction time/reflexes are exceptionally slow, or they can't feel below their knees due to neuropathy, then they likely shouldn't be driving, and I have a duty to report those findings.

When discussing a physical or functional decline, I usually review the overall current status of the patient and then explore the particular goals of the individual. There is a discussion regarding the possible, realistic, future state. This requires a high degree of motivation which includes knowing the interests of the patient, the patient's current ability and desire to improve the quality of life. The patience required to see an increase in their exercise capacity and hitting barriers such as plateaus or injuries also needs to be explored. I also try and gauge what has and has not worked in the past, when I review the success or failure outcomes from past attempts at health-related goal setting. Of all these factors, motivation is key. There are no current medications to prescribe, to increase motivation, otherwise I'd be taking them. Most people fail at health-related goals due to emotional factors that interfere with success. Often, this is due to acknowledged or subliminal self sabotage. It is here that I often see the self-fulfilling prophecy come to life. I see this often when an individual of any age or health status, joins a gym or a new weight loss group. Sometimes the goal setting for these tasks is too large, too broad, unrealistic, and unattainable. As the saying goes … "How do you eat an elephant?" The answer is one bite at a time. This is the premise of SMART goal setting where the goals reflect breaking up an activity or goal into smaller, more attainable goals. This is the most common step-wise approach that I use both personally and with coaching clients. No plan is complete without a clear destination and timeline for the desired state. If I was on a driving vacation and didn't have a clear road map, I would never achieve the goal of where my vacation was supposed to take me. This is why maps are required for trip planning. With a clear, time sensitive plan of how to increase the activities expanded upon in this book and by improving fitness and functionality, then the result of less frailty, will be achieved and hopefully, successful aging in place can continue.

As a health care provider or family member, be the elder person's accountability partner, if they don't already have one. Develop together, a clear plan and time sensitive approach using the information in the following chapters. Be sure to align the plan with the goals as **prioritized by the senior** you are assisting. The elderly individual must prioritize what is most important to him/her/them before anyone else can help achieve those goals. Family members, allied health profession-als, nurses, nurse practitioners, and physicians are there to encourage success and not dwell on an individual's failure. The exploration of perceived failures can often re invigorate and re motivate a client to work differently to achieve the next goal. Accountability partners need to be there to help the individual acknowledge how things got derailed. Once the issues have been identified and alternate plans are created, then the partners goal is to help motivate the senior to attempt these important modified tasks again. For example, when weight loss has not been achieved, there should be no fat shaming. The accountability partner should focus on what has gone well (better eating habits, more stamina, regular bowel movements, and other benefits). These unintended consequences that need to be highlighted and celebrated, rather than focusing on the lack of weight loss. This is where life coaching may be beneficial. Sometimes an outside professional can help people get out of their own way by exploring the role of self sabotage and other negative influences, that are impairing the achievement of certain goals. Fitness trainers, private physiotherapists, and kinesiologists can all have a role in getting the tasks done as well. But it must be an established priority of the senior to achieve those goals, before other professionals can be brought in to assist in supporting roles. There is often a financial cost for these services so motivation to pay for this assistance is absolutely required, before other team members can be brought into the program.

What about health-care providers? How can they help with their patients? I feel our primary role as clinicians, is to provide up to date education about the risk benefit ratios of proposed medications, activities, procedures, and treatments. Not all caregivers are comfortable with providing exercise prescriptions, but this book gives everyone some basic guidelines to initiate the exercise prescription process. All programs should be individualized over time. There needs to be an expectation of progression for frailty to diminish, as well as clear instructions on when to stop activities and seek out medical attention if any symptoms occur with activity.

As a child of one remaining elderly parent, I also have put my money where my mouth is. All the bed, brain, resistance, balance, and cardio exercises have been performed on a regular basis by myself since researching the concepts in this book. My father, due to severe medical illnesses and immobility, can not do many of the resistance, balance, or cardio portions of this book, but he has participated in the brain training exercises denoted in Chapter 7. I don't have a gym membership or nor have I invested in expensive exercise equipment. I have chosen to use easily available/inexpensive equipment such as resistance tubing, small barbells, my own body weight, my workout partner, empty milk jugs, cans of soup and many other available items at home. This is why I advocate for developing an activity routine in the safety of your own home, to be done at any time of the day which suits the individual trying to achieve a fitness goal.

And while I do many of these activities daily, I believe in setting an example yourself is critical to engaging your loved ones to follow suit. This way, you won't be saying "Do what I say, not what I do." Transparency and the belief in modelling these important activities is key to successfully engaging your loved ones to mirror your behaviour.

CHAPTER SUMMARY

This chapter outlines the basic triad of factors required to successfully age in place. If physical and cognitive fitness and functionality are not maintained in the fifties, sixties, seventies, and eighties, then one or both of the other two factors, family and finances will need to be in abundance in order for seniors to safely age in place.

CHAPTER 4:
ESSENTIALS OF EXERCISE PRESCRIPTIONS AND CARDIAC REHABILITATION

Some people want it to happen, some wish it would happen, others make it happen. —Michael Jordan

After twenty-five years of cardiac exercise testing, the most consistent and enlightening information that clients receive after having a stress test is—realizing that they're not as fit as they thought they were. I have many clients who come for stress testing, usually because they have chest pain or other cardiorespiratory symptoms that require investigations to rule out cardiac disease as an etiology for their symptoms. I had the exceptional opportunity to work at an outstanding public/private cardiac rehabilitation facility in Manitoba.[21] This was the ideal mix of public and private services. It was a public-pay gym membership for those people who didn't have any cardiac disease. If desired, members could self-pay for cardiac stress testing, to assist in developing a safe exercise regimen. The other mix of clients at that facility, were the folks who had already had some sort of vascular event. This could be a heart attack, stents, bypass surgery, artificial heart valve surgery, arrhythmia diagnosis, new onset congestive heart failure and stroke. After an encounter in the health care system, the clients would be referred post-discharge from any of the surrounding clinics or hospitals. Part of their rehabilitation program was funded, but there was also a fee for each attendee to complete the cardiac rehabilitation educational and exercise prescription program.

The goal of the program was to provide education and lifestyle skills and exercise prescriptions in order to decrease the risk of having another vascular event (secondary prevention).

Cardiac rehabilitation is one of the best prescriptions clinicians can offer clients for improving quality of life and secondary prevention.

---

21 https://www.reh-fit.com/

When clients are referred for secondary prevention, there's a component of overall cardiovascular assessment (history and physical exam), objective assessment of exercise risk and tolerance (graded exercise tolerance test or treadmill test), and specialist overview as deemed necessary by the multidisciplinary team (specialists volunteered their time after clinics). Ongoing regular assessment and progress of the members, specifically in their response to their individualized exercise prescription, occurred with every interaction. There was also a component of team troubleshooting, should any new symptoms or events have occurred while the clients were exercising. This was all performed in a setting where specially trained resuscitative staff could embark upon life saving measures (medications, defibrillator, CPR, and full cardiac arrest care) should there be any unexpected cardiac events in any of the members. Unlike the majority of health care provided by myself in the past, I found this work environment to be extremely motivating and rewarding, as everyone was participating without coercion, to prevent the next cardiovascular event. It was every member's goal to successfully improve their own personal fitness and functional level. The social interactions at the walking track and educational sessions, fitness rooms, all combined with a high level of qualified care givers providing care, education, and psychological debriefing, provided an unparalleled level of socialization, peer support and counselling unlike most other clinics. There was the common thread of surviving cardiovascular disease and all members were universally supportive of each other in the programs. The members looked out for one another and reported concerns to the staff. Some friendship bonds lasted many years. For me, this was one of the most rewarding work environments I had ever encountered and I still believe this program is unparalleled in any of my work experiences in the last several decades. When I went to that facility to work, I never had to convince any of the clients regarding the need to exercise, diet, or prioritize themselves. For once in their lives, these clients had started to prioritize themselves and felt very fortunate that they had survived the most frightening event in their lives to date. Sometimes these folks developed a post traumatic stress disorder, especially if they had cardiac bypass surgery or a very complicated hospital course. Fortunately, psychologists and counsellors were also available to deal with these psychological issues.

With regards to exercise stress testing programs, almost every Canadian facility uses the standard "Bruce protocol" of exercise, which has been around for one hundred years. It's been standardized so that the incline and speed of the treadmill change every three minutes. There are certainly other protocols such as modified Bruce, Naughton, and other protocols that are utilized in clients who aren't active enough for the standard Bruce protocol.

I'm a big believer in exercise stress testing prior to giving somebody an exercise prescription. This is the ultimate gold standard. But within Canadian remote and rural settings, and even busy urban clinics, this is a relatively limited resource, and not everyone can get this test done. In training, we're taught not to do testing if the pre-test probability of an illness is low.[22] Some private clinics offer stress testing services for a fee, paid for by the individual client themselves. I can't reiterate how much important information I get from these tests, but I'm not certain everyone needs to pay out of pocket for this type of screening before exercise is prescribed if some common ground rules are followed. These ground rules will be explored later in the chapter.

Are there options in Canada to pay privately for this testing?[23,24,25] While there are some opportunities for private pay assessments, a client must look carefully at the cost benefit ratio for this type of service. There are always false positive and false negative tests. What is the individual willing to do if a false positive test occurs? How is the health care system set up to deal with these issues? Both of these questions are complicated and beyond the scope of this book.

---

22 Vieira, Alexandre R; "Pre-test Probabilities and Test Selection in Population Screening and Diagnosis"; Journal of Medical Decision Making; March 2020

23 "How Much Does a Private ECG-Exercise (or Stress) Cost in the UK?" Private Healthcare UK, accessed August 23, 2022, https://www.privatehealth.co.uk/conditions-and-treatments/ecg-exercise-or-stress/costs/.

24 "Ottawa Private Medical Clinic Offers 5-Hour, $1,200 Checkup," CBC, January 15, 2008, https://www.cbc.ca/news/canada/ottawa/ottawa-private-medical-clinic-offers-5-hour-1-200-checkup-1.708173.

25 False Creek Wellness, https://www.falsecreekdiagnostics.com/.

During the test, the patient is hooked up to a twelve-lead electrocardiogram, modifying the leads so that they aren't on the arms and legs, which will be moving with exercise (this reduces the "artifact" or muscle interference with interpreting the cardiac waveforms). The goal of any stress test is to get the patient to do some physical activity while monitored. Clinicians ideally want clients to try and achieve their target heart rate (THR). Maximum (100 percent) age-appropriate target heart rate is 220 subtract current age. In order to do a cardiac workload, we expect people to be able to do 80–90 percent of their age-appropriate maximum heart rate. The useful information obtained from this test includes resting heart rate, blood pressure, and resting electrocardiogram. We get a sense of exercise tolerance by looking at the heart rate and blood pressure response to the degree of exercise and how quickly one achieves THR. We look for the presence of inducible arrhythmias with exercise. We review the symptoms that clients have with exertion and see if those symptoms can be reproduced while exercising on the treadmill. If symptoms are reproduced, the clinician will try and correlate those symptoms with ECG or rhythm abnormalities. This test is done under the supervision with both cardiology technologists and an appropriately trained physician. These tests occur in locations where there is an ability to perform life saving interventions should an arrhythmia or other cardiac event occur. The results are available immediately and the physician will determine whether additional studies are required (in the event of a positive or inconclusive test). Although it's not a perfect test in men and women (for different reasons), the stress test can usually clear a client for an immediate and safe exercise prescription. The other benefit is that there is no exposure to radiation or dyes with a plain exercise stress test.

I pay particular attention in making the client aware of when they are in their target heart rate zone. This is when they get into the 80–90 percent range of the age-predicted maximum, and I usually point out the target heart rate range by asking the client to reflect upon the degree of perceived exertion that they are currently experiencing at the time of achieving THR. If clients are working "hard to very hard" they are almost always in their THR range (80 to 90 percent of age-predicted heart rate maximum). The exceptions would be those clients who are severely deconditioned or have other illnesses such as COPD or arrhythmias. I then educate the client on how long it took to achieve THR on the treadmill when they get to the THR zone. If the information is available, I compare the client's progress to that of age-related normal clients. The test is completed when the client has symptoms, achieves target heart rate for more 1-3 minutes, or is unable to do any further workload. In the recovery/resting period, which can range from four to ten minutes, clinicians continuously review the ECG as it returns to normal. The Cardiology technologist and the physician look at heart rate recovery - how long it takes for the heart rate to get under 100 bpm from maximum exercise. The staff will also review any arrhythmias (if present) and how the blood pressure recovers from the workload.

The physician will then make a summary of whether or not the test is clinically (symptoms present) or electrocardiographically (ECG changes or arrhythmias present) positive. The physician will also ideally comment on the fitness level of the individual and suggest or make arrangements to do additional testing if indicated. Sometimes, advice regarding medication management is given if needed. This might include adding a blood pressure agent or changing the angina or heart failure medications. This is an individual clinician dependent decision and varies from practitioner to practitioner. The supervising physician may also give the client an exercise prescription based on how the client did at the time of the treadmill test.

Most clients are only in their target heart rate zone for two to three minutes during the stress test. The client is usually shocked by the limited time they were able to tolerate this ideal heart rate during the test. Clinicians get enough information by keeping the client in the target heart rate zone for that small duration of time, and at the end of the test, I explain that all adults need to have 150 to 300 minutes per week of exercise within that target heart rate zone. This is an eye opener for almost all patients!

The 150 weekly minute prescription is a *minimum* quantity of target heart rate exercise, which equates to thirty minutes in target heart rate zone at least five days per week. Not included in that thirty minutes is the mandatory five-minute warmup and a five-to-ten-minute cool down. Clients are unanimously shocked to acknowledge the amount of workload required to be considered as cardiovascular fitness.

The exercise prescription I provide for the client is to initiate exercise a day after their stress test and make it a daily exercise regimen. They need to start every session with a five-minute warmup, slowly increasing their heart rate to get into their target heart rate zone for three to five minutes on their first day, and then every day or two, increase the duration of time in the target heart rate zone by one to two minutes. By the time clients have done this five days a week for a month, they should be at the level of 150 minutes of exercise in the target heart rate zone per week. While one might be tempted to accelerate the exercise program sooner than this, injuries often occur when warmups don't take place, and the progress is too fast for the client's fitness level.

I also explain that if your heart is healthy, you should be able to slowly increase your workload. If you can't, this may imply the need for further testing, and individuals will need to liaise with their primary care provider to see if additional testing is required. I also advise clients not to try and push their workload faster than instructed. The slow, orderly, and gradual increase in activity is safer and will help prevent injuries. It's a very methodical way of increasing your cardiac workload, but within one month's time, most clients will achieve their THR goal and 150 minutes per week as their minimal exercise goal (see below on stress testing limitations).

As we age, we need less of a heart rate to gain cardiac benefits with exercise. The eighty-five percent THR is for "healthy individuals" in the age group who successfully and incrementally can increase the activity without the development of injuries or concerning symptoms (fainting, light-headedness, chest pain, profound shortness of breath, palpitations, or other worrisome/new symptoms). If you're not sure about your health, then you can start using the seventy percent target heart rate range until you successfully exercise for more than one month. Then weekly, if no symptoms occur, you can increase your THR by five percent per week until you're at your eighty-five percent THR goal.

The chart below highlights the *eighty-five percent THR* for most *presumably healthy clients*, and the *seventy percent range* is where I suggest starting, for those clients with recent heart attacks (wait six weeks or as directed by cardiologist), known congestive heart failure, recent surgery (need surgeon clearance and wait at least six weeks), and severe deconditioning/frailty.

I have organized some of these thoughts in the chart below to assist clients in determining how to proceed, especially if one does not have access to primary health care. The balance and resistance training will be elaborated upon in other chapters in the book.

EXERCISE CHART INCLUDING TARGET HEART RATE RANGE IN AGE GROUPS FOR RELATIVELY HEALTHY CLIENTS AND IMPAIRED HEALTH OR HIGH-RISK FACTORS FOR HEART DISEASE IN CLIENTS

AGE	THR (220-AGE) MAX HR	85% THR Presumed healthy	70% THR* Unsure of health status or known cardiac conditions	STRESS TEST REQUIRED?	BALANCE EXERCISES	LIGHT RESISTANCE TRAINING	CAVEATS
50–59	161–170	136–145	112–119	NOT LIKELY	YES	YES	If available, always check in with your primary care provider
50–59*			112–119	IDEALLY	YES	YES	1
60–69	151–160	128–136	106–112	NOT LIKELY	YES	YES	2
60–69*			106–112	IDEALLY	YES	YES	3
70–79	141–150	120–127	99–105	IDEALLY	YES	YES	4
70–79*			99–105	IDEALLY	YES	YES	5
80–89	131–140	111–119	78–83	IDEALLY	YES	YES	6
80–89*			78–83	IDEALLY	YES	YES	7
90+	<130	<110	<91	POSSIBLY*	YES	POSSIBLY*	8
90+*			<91	POSSIBLY*	YES	POSSIBLY*	9, 10, 11

*THOSE CLIENTS WITH PRE-EXISTING HEART DISEASE, ANGINA, CHF, COPD, or VERY DECONDITIONED/OUT OF SHAPE/COUCH POTATO/ NEWCOMER TO EXERCISE

Below I have included the New York Heart Association classification for heart failure symptoms that help clinicians guide medical management, including goal-directed medical therapy for heart failure or other chronic diseases. It also gives the average person the knowledge to review one's symptoms when exercising.

Those clients who have heart disease, congestive heart failure, uncontrolled hypertension, activity triggered angina, all need to do a basic NYHA class assessment before proceeding to exercise. _The symptoms are fatigue, palpitations, chest pain, dyspnea (shortness of breath), and syncope (or loss of consciousness)._

Those who are in NYHA class I can continue with their exercise program using the lower target heart rate of seventy percent unless directed by their physician or specialist to achieve a THR of eighty-five percent.

Clients who have NYHA class II or III symptoms can certainly exercise as per the NYHA class I clients, but at a reduced workload or time commitment, as long as symptoms don't accelerate quickly or change from your prior workouts.

Clients who have NYHA class III symptoms, or if their symptoms are progressing or accelerating, may choose to attempt their usual exercise program, or reduce the THR by five to ten percent from the last workout. They may change their activities to include stationary biking instead of walking, chair exercises instead of standing exercises, or just working on their balance and range of motion if their symptoms are getting worse. Of course, seeking medical attention for a possible change in medications or possibly other interventions may be required.

NYHA class IV symptoms give one a severe inability to do almost any activity in the home. In this case, exercise with resistance training or cardio exercise regimens should be _avoided_ until reviewed by your primary care provider or specialist. Ideally, these clients would exercise only in supervised cardiac rehabilitations type settings. If you develop new onset NYHA class IV symptoms, you may need to go to the emergency room for an immediate assessment if your symptoms are new, progressive, or unexpected.

If you have angina (chest pain with exertion) and experience some symptoms of chest pain at a certain workload, you may continue your workload at a lower level by choosing a target heart rate that is 10 bpm below the threshold that gives you angina. But again, you should stop the work out until you are cleared by your practitioner.

If you have new onset angina with your usual workload, or you notice a progressive activity intolerance over the last few exercise sessions, you should no longer exercise until you can seek out medical attention, as you may require further risk assessment, testing, and/or medication adjustments.

Caveats

Review these if you have any conditions that cause you to question the safety of exercise.

- 1= severe osteoarthritis. Arthritis affects about twenty-four percent of adults in the US. Fifty-six percent of older men and sixty-nine percent of older women aged sixty-five and older. Hip and knee osteoarthritis are most prevalent, and muscle weakness is considered a modifiable primary risk factor for knee pain, disability, and progression of joint damage. Those folks with advanced osteoarthritis and even rheumatoid arthritis, can experience considerable gains in muscle strength after resistance training, without resulting increases in pain or other ill effects.
- 2= chronic kidney disease (CKD). CKD affects up to forty-six percent of the older population in the United States, compared with fourteen percent of the general population. Chronic kidney disease related muscle wasting is associated with loss of muscle strength and impaired functional status or physical functioning, which is progressive. Protein calorie malnutrition, protein degradation, hormone resistance in muscle building hormones, and many chronic inflammatory markers can make muscle weakness and wasting substantially worse. Inflammatory cytokines and impaired insulin and other hormone signaling from inflammation, chronic metabolic

acidosis, and other hormones that stimulate protein destruction, all result in continued muscle wasting. Resistance exercise provides a variety of benefits to those with CKD, including increased albumin, increased muscle strength, increased physical functionality, possibly increased GFR, reduced inflammation, improved muscle function, increased skeletal muscle growth, increased muscular strength, and improved quality of life. Adequate volume status, blood sugar, and blood pressure control are necessary in this CKD group who are working on increasing their resistance training or doing any aerobic exercise regimen.

- 3= osteoporosis. The prevalence of this condition is one in twelve is adults age sixty to sixty-nine, and one in four adults over eighty. It's a painful, and often debilitating condition, that contributes to impaired health-related quality of life. Resistance training can be beneficial by increasing bone mineral content, preventing fall related fractures, significantly improving physical function, pain, and quality of life. The resistance exercise program needs to be tailored so that the presence of pain is treated and tolerable, and most programs require a lower intensity and slower rate of progression.

- 4= obesity. There is an increasing prevalence of obesity in North America. In the US, approximately thirty-nine percent of adults are obese, but there is wide variability across different populations. Obesity has significant pathophysiologic consequences on both bone and skeletal muscle health and function. Infiltration of the muscles with fatty material, excessive visceral adiposity (belly fat), increases in the infiltration of lipids (fatty tissue) in non-adipose organs (liver or skeletal muscle) and is more common in type 2 diabetes. Prolonged sedentary behavior combined with adipose site–derived hormones, cytokines, and inflammation lead to increased muscle weakness which is referred to as sarcopenic obesity. The excessive adiposity (increased fat tissue) in obese older adults would create a double negative effect of not only having an increased overall body mass, but also a decreased ability for that person to lift their mass, due to a reduced quality of muscle. Resistance training needs to be added to general physical activity, cardiorespiratory exercise, and a multidisciplinary approach is required to deal with this complex disease process. Medications for obesity will be touched upon in another chapter. As an adult with refractory obesity, I am most keen on helping obese patients reduce the risk of obesity related sarcopenia and other obesity related complications.

- 5= uncontrolled hypertension (possibly aortic root dilatation and/or thoracic chronic aortic dissections). These conditions can affect a significant portion of the elderly population. Acute elevations of blood pressure or poorly controlled hypertension, are contraindications to exercise and resistance exercises, until the blood pressure is under control and being managed by a primary care provider. Resistance training needs to progress at a much slower rate and a lower resistance level to avoid exercised-induced elevations in blood pressure. Valsalva manoeuvres (bearing down like when you want to have a bowel movement or bearing down when lifting weights) should be avoided at all costs in this group, and a more prolonged cool down period may be required to avoid potential hypotensive episodes after abrupt cessation of activity

- 6= congestive heart failure. Exercise improves skeletal muscle atrophy. Cardiac weight and muscle loss, may be improved with increased exercise capacity and resistance training. There has to be a lack of clinical symptoms at rest, absence of postural hypotension (difference between lying and standing blood pressures), absence of known pulmonary or venous congestion (dyspnea, weight gain, increased swelling), stable weight, stable kidney function, and stable electrolytes (sodium, potassium, and magnesium) before resistance training can be entertained. Heart failure clients tend to have an exaggerated respiratory rate response to exercise. Therefore, shortness of breath will limit exercise tolerance.

- 7= cognitive impairment. The choice of exercises will need to be simple and may require extra instruction and demonstration. Overall, exercise is VERY BENEFICIAL for cognitive decline or dementia.
- 8= visually impaired, low back pain or balance issues. Consider using weight machines as opposed to free weights to reduce the risk of injury to the client.
- 9= mobility conditions. Safety is the main priority, and starting with exercises modified for the seated position will be safer and better tolerated in the beginning of an exercise program.
- 10= frailty. We will need to modify our program to start at a lower resistance, progress more slowly, and limit the endpoint to well short of complete fatigue.
- 11= COPD or lung disease. See Chapter 5 for further details.

Now that we have explored the two basic exercise regimens for people who believe they are healthy versus those who have known medical conditions or are severely deconditioned (out of shape), you may ask, "Why are clinicians so big on promoting exercise?" In this next section, I'll go through some of the literature that's available that speaks about the evidence regarding exercise programs, not only for cardiovascular benefit but also for frailty prevention.

Exercise to reduce your risk of major illnesses such as coronary artery disease, stroke, type 2 diabetes, and cancer can also lower your risk of early death by up to thirty percent. It's free, has an immediate effect and most[26] of us don't need to seek out medical attention before we start a gentle exercise program. I'm not saying that we should all go and start training for a marathon! On the contrary, I'm asking that all adults engage in a slowly progressive program that gets to the minimum required activity of 150 minutes per week along with resistance training, balance training, and brain training. The latter three will be explored in future chapters.

---

26 Please consult with your primary care provider if you have any concerns about starting an exercise program!

While the overall role of exercises is known to be beneficial, it can also assist people with many conditions as outlined in the caveat section of the above table. Exercise needs to be individualized and patient-centred, taking into account factors such as age, mobility, pain, and other comorbidities.[27]

Regarding frailty and the development of sarcopenia, exercise along with resistance training has been shown to have anti-inflammatory effects and may reduce the progression to frailty. There is an increasing amount of evidence that proves that exercise is good in all age groups and in all levels of physical ability, including disability, stroke, and even bedridden patients.[28]

In weight management, the role of exercise is also very important, but it alone won't promote weight loss unless one is exercising greater than three hundred minutes per week in the target heart rate range of eighty-five percent or higher. Physical activity is still recommended for all patients who are overweight,[29] and strength training will help prevent the sarcopenia of obesity, which further accelerates frailty.

Next, I will outline a basic exercise/cardio (#1) regimen for adults who feel well, have no significant health issues, and feel that they can start a gentle workload without additional training. If you have any difficulties with symptoms that seem out of proportion to the workload you are doing, stop immediately and refrain from further training until you've been checked out by your primary care provider, Urgent Care Centre, or Emergency Room at the local hospital. If you develop any chest pain that does not immediately go away with stopping the activity, call 911.

---

27 Kim L. Bennell and Rana S. Hinman, "A Review of the Clinical Evidence for Exercise in Osteoarthritis of the Hip and Knee," accessed August 23, 2022, http://www.yhep.com.au/documents/JSAMS-Article-Osteoarthritis-of-the-hip-and-knee1.pdf.

28 Stephen C. Allen, "Systemic Inflammation in the Genesis of Frailty and Sarcopenia: An Overview of the Preventative and Therapeutic Role of Exercise and the Potential for Drug Treatments," Geriatrics, January 17, 2017, https://mdpi-res.com/d_attachment/geriatrics/geriatrics-02-00006/article_deploy/geriatrics-02-00006.pdf.

29 Damon L. Swift, Neil M. Johannsen, et al, "The Role of Exercise and Physical Activity in Weight Loss and Management," National Library of Medicine, January 1, 2015, https://www.ncbi.nlm.nih.gov/pmc/articles/PMC3925973/.

EXERTION SCALES

It is important to gauge how well an individual is tolerating the workload being attempted. Here is a simple exertion scale with 0 being no exertion whatsoever, to 10 which is maximum exertion and **not** the recommended goal of activity. Ideally, the scale should be 6-8 with episodes of achieving 9 if progressive cardiovascular fitness goals are being prescribed.

Level	Examples of Activity	Heart Rate	I feel like …
0	resting, sleep deprived, jet lagged, comatose from imbibing in too many spirits	variable	Oh my God, I'm so exhausted; opening my eyes is challenging; going to the bathroom at a turtle's pace.
1	making coffee, feeding the cat, limited slow walking short distances	60–70	I am so tired and my movements are slow and sloth-like!
2	I need to climb a few stairs to go get cat food from the basement.	70–80	I think I'll store the cat food upstairs.
3	slow walking at a normal pace	80–90	I can do this for hours!
4	moderate walking speed or small inclines	90–100	I can do this for an hour.
5	walking like you're late for school/ appointment for a sustained period of time	100–110	I'm huffing and puffing but can carry on a conversation; I can do this for forty-five minutes.
6	periodic high intensity interval train-ing: one power walk for five minutes and then stop and do twenty-five jumping jacks to get HR elevated	110–120	I can do this for another half hour or so.
7	Sweet spot: I am working quite hard and feel good about the performance.	110–130	Endorphins are being released; I am experiencing a "runner's high" but I can only say two to three words at a time; I still have five minutes left in me at this pace.
8	Sweet spot: I am at my target heart rate and can continue on for only a short while.	130–140	Can't talk much, have only one to two minutes left at this level; I would die if a bear presented itself right now.
9	Sub maximal effort: no need to work this hard unless training for a marathon	140–155	Can't talk; have less than one minute in reserve.
10	Maximum effort	155+	Oh my God! I'm going to die if I don't stop now.

BASIC CARDIO EXERCISE PRESCRIPTION #1

* If *healthy*/no heart disease/CHF/uncontrolled hypertension/etc.

	Warm up	Target heart rate (85%) Minutes per session in THR zone	EXERTION SCALE	Progression (pace = walking like you're late for an appointment)	Cool down	Frequency	Incline If using treadmill
Week 1	5 mins	3–5	4-6	Increase THR by 1–2 minutes each session	5 mins	3Xweek	0
Week 2	5 mins	11–21	4-6	Increase THR 1– 2 mins per session	5–6 mins	5Xweek	0
Week 3	5 min	21–25	4-7	Increase THR 1–2 minutes per session	6–7 mins	5Xweek	0
Week 4	5 mins	25–35	5-7	At THR time; increase duration if weight loss required	10 mins	5Xweek	0
Week 5-8	5 mins	30–35	6-8	At THR time; increase duration if weight loss required	10 mins	5Xweek	3–5% grade
Week 9–12	5 mins	30–35	6-8	At THR time; increase duration if weight loss required	10 mins	5Xweek	5–10% grade
Week 12+	5 mins	30–35	6-9	At THR time; increase duration if weight loss required	10 mins	5Xweek	10% + as desired

The next chart will outline a basic exercise/cardio (#2) regimen for adults who are deconditioned, not used to exercising, or have significant health issues but feel that they can start a gentle workload at this time. If you have any difficulties with symptoms that seem out of proportion to the workload you are doing, stop immediately and refrain from further training until you've been checked out by your primary care provider, Urgent Care Centre, or Emergency Room at the local hospital. If you develop any chest pain that does not immediately go away with stopping the activity, call 911.

BASIC CARDIO EXERCISE PRESCRIPTION #2

* If unhealthy/deconditioned/out of shape/heart disease/CHF/uncontrolled hypertension etc.

	Warm up	Target heart rate (70%) Minutes per session in THR zone	EXERTIONAL SCALE 1-10	Progression (pace = walking like you're late for an appointment)	Cool down	Frequency	Incline If using treadmill
Week 1	5 mins	3–5	2-3	Increase THR by ½–1 min each session	5 mins	3Xweek	0
Week 2	5 mins	5–11	2-3	Increase THR ½–1 min per session	5–6 mins	5Xweek	0
Week 3	5 min	11–18	3-4	Increase THR ½–1 min per session	6–7 mins	5Xweek	0
Week 4	5 mins	18–23	3-4	Increase THR ½–1 min per session	10 mins	5Xweek	0
Week 5–8	5 mins	23–28	4-6	Increase THR ½–1 min per session	10 mins	5Xweek	0
Week 9–12	5 mins	28–32	4-6	Increase THR ½–1 min per session	10 mins	5Xweek	1–4% grade
Week 12+	5 mins	>30	5-7	At 150 mins per week	10 mins	5Xweek	5% + as desired/tolerated

I don't always often suggest tracking with a Fitbit or Apple watch unless the client already has those items purchased. Over the years, I've found that the perceived exertion scale gives people an idea of their target heart rate when they're working out. Very light to somewhat hard (4-6) is for patients who have heart disease or congestive heart failure, and hard to very hard (8-9) is for most of the other clients.

Dr. Karen's Exertional Scale 1-10

Level	Examples of Activity	Heart Rate	I feel like …
0	resting, sleep deprived, jet lagged, comatose from imbibing, dead	60	Oh my God, I'm so exhausted; opening my eyes is challenging; going to the bathroom at a turtle's pace.
1	making coffee, feeding the cat, limited slow walking short distances	60–70	I am so tired and my movements are slow and sloth-like!
2	I need to climb a few stairs to go get cat food from the basement.	70–80	I think I'll store the cat food upstairs.
3	slow walking at a normal pace	80–90	I can do this for hours!
4	moderate walking speed or small inclines	90–100	I can do this for an hour.
5	walking like you're late for school/appointment for a sustained period of time	100–110	I'm huffing and puffing but can carry on a conversation; I can do this for forty-five minutes.
6	periodic high intensity interval training: one power walk for five minutes and then stop and do twenty-five jumping jacks to get HR elevated	110–120	I can do this for another half hour or so.
7	Sweet spot: I am working quite hard and feel good about the performance.	110–130	Endorphins are being released; I am experiencing a "runner's high" but I can only say two to three words at a time; I still have five minutes left in me at this pace.
8	Sweet spot: I am at my target heart rate and can continue on for only a short while.	130–140	Can't talk much, have only one to two minutes left at this level; I would die if a bear presented itself right now.
9	Sub maximal effort: no need to work this hard unless training for a marathon	140–155	Can't talk; have less than one minute in reserve.
10	Maximum effort	155+	Oh my God! I'm going to die if I don't stop now.

As clients do their activities of daily living or low-grade workouts, I'd like them to note where they are on the perceived exertion scale. Certainly, if light housework is a 7-8, then that individual will want to go quite slow when starting other activities. If another client can lift drywall and hold it in place while securing the drywall to walls, and they perceive this exertion as 3, then this individual can likely be a little more aggressive in starting his or her exercise program.

Look to see where you are on the exertion scale when you do your household tasks today.

CHAPTER SUMMARY

In this chapter, we've reviewed the basics of cardiac exercise testing and the two basic exercise prescriptions for people who are relatively fit and/or healthy (#1) versus those who are extremely unfit or with significant comorbid conditions (#2).

Overall, the benefits of exercise in older adults includes increased mobility, enhanced performance of activities of daily living, improved gait, decreased falls, improved bone mineral density, and increased general well-being. Numerous articles in the medical literature support these concepts. Studies suggest that even the older, frailest adults are likely to benefit from physical activity at almost any level that can be safely tolerated. While some clients will never meet the recommended targets, even modest activity with reduced intensity and durations and muscle training can slow the progression of functional limitations. Improved functionality will allow us to stay in our own homes, in a safer environment, for a longer period of time, if we just initiate this inexpensive (exercise can be done anywhere) and critically important treatment in any willing adult's plan of care.

CHAPTER 5:
ESSENTIALS OF RESPIRATORY REHABILITATION PROGRAMS

The last chapter focused on the essentials of cardiac rehabilitation and exercise prescriptions. This chapter will focus on those individuals with known or unknown respiratory conditions that may prevent the individual from fully participating in an exercise program. In clinic, I often see clients in the clinic who have grown older but have never participated in a regular exercise regimen. When discussing the benefits of exercise, a great deal of clients acknowledge that exercise could be beneficial but most will find almost any excuse to not exercise. Again, I find that people either like or dislike exercise, and trying to convince somebody who has never exercised in their life to change their behaviour is extremely challenging! What's even more challenging is convincing the older adult who continues to smoke cigarettes (and/or other substances) to both quit smoking and start exercising. These folks have never had to exercise because the nicotine in the tobacco often keeps the clients within a tolerable body weight and attempts at quitting smoking in the past has resulted in weight gain. These are some of the more challenging groups to convince that tobacco cessation and exercise programs are essential for long-term health. A paternalistic "physician knows best" attitude is rarely successful in getting the client to change these behaviours, habits, and patterns. While I have been a healthcare provider for many years, my training as a coach has enlightened me more on assisting clients to "buy in" to recommended therapies. Behaviour change meetings are not isolated consultations. Behaviour changes require ongoing meeting after trust with the coach or care giver has been established. This is where the coach is accepted as an accountability and thought partner with the client. Together, this team can explore the barriers getting in the way of a client's success. In our current health care models, most primary care clinicians don't have the time available to truly do this coaching job justice (continued coaching and reinforcement with accountability planning). Thus, clients and clinicians both need to explore other team members available to provide this critical "coaching" service. In primary care models such as Community Health Centres (CHCs), this may be a more successful strategy as there are many team members who can participate in this coaching program. The data about successes in this type of care setting is currently lacking but in theory, it is likely a very beneficial model for clients who need lifestyle behaviour modification for overall health. There may also be a role to play for privately funded "home care services" or life coach services, where the client can pay for this type of education, accountability, and behavioural reinforcement. Again, health care and outcome data will be required to recommend any of these programs going forward.

The respiratory care of our aging populations is very important. At our current time in health care history, most primary care clinics are not concerned with population health, nor are they concerned with climate change and the resultant population health changes. Given the clinician resource dilemma, clinicians focus on practicing individual client care. I am pleased that governments are moving toward the concepts of alternative models of health care like CHCs (Community Health Centres). One of the mandates of the CHC is to review the ability to provide "population-based care" especially to catchment areas where access to primary care is limited. In my experience, population care programs will be a much needed resource for some of these chronic illnesses in the population.

I feel that respiratory diseases could be one of the population-based care programs to be developed and promoted. This is due to the statistics of chronic lung disease in Canada. Of the over 38 million people who live in Canada, it's believed that 3 million have COPD (chronic obstructive pulmonary disease). About 1.5 million people are aware of their diagnosis, and an equal number have no knowledge of their disease. The diagnosis of chronic lung disease relies on recognizing symptoms and seeking out medical care for those symptoms. Ideally, confirmatory pulmonary function tests that show obstruction or hyperinflation are performed to solidify the diagnosis. In addition to chronic OBSTRUCTIVE lung disease, there are many other forms of lung disease which may result in similar symptoms. In addition to the prevalence of known and occult lung disease in Canada, we are also bombarded by the climate changes that contribute to phenomena such as intolerable heat domes and wild fires contributing to unhealthy ambient air.

When reviewing formal pulmonary rehabilitation programs, the success of programs has been based on improving the symptoms and activity tolerance of COPD clients. This chapter will focus on some of the details of those programs. But due to lack of access to these programs for the majority of patients, I wish to educate the adults in our population about those basic concepts of respiratory care, especially if you do not have access to a primary care provider. The overall activity plans that I have created can include those folks with known or unknown respiratory conditions. These programs include balance exercises, low resistance weight training, and low-level cardio which will be beneficial for those clients with and without pulmonary disease. This chapter will review the basics of a pulmonary rehabilitation program but just like cardiac rehabilitation and exercise prescriptions, pulmonary rehabilitation also needs to be individualized for each client. And just like cardiac rehabilitation, what should you do if access to these beneficial programs is non existent?

While pulmonary rehabilitation can improve the respiratory symptoms, pulmonary function, quality of life, and healthcare utilization, it may also improve overall lifespan in those with COPD. COPD includes a mix of one, two or three main symptoms. One is that of chronic bronchitis, where clients present with a chronic cough or sputum production. The second aspect is that of hyper reactivity in the airways where wheezing may occur. The third component is that of emphysema where there are anatomical disruptions of the small air sacs in the lungs, where oxygen transfer occurs.[30] Smoking not only increases the risk of COPD but also increases the risk of cancer.

---

30 "COPD," Mayo Clinic, accessed August 23, 2022, https://www.mayoclinic.org/
   diseases-conditions/copd/symptoms-causes/syc-20353679.

The most important goal for friends, families, and caregivers of clients who smoke, is promoting successful cessation of tobacco and nicotine use (and any other smoked substance as well). Once this is accomplished, other therapeutic treatments, such as oxygen therapy, bronchodilators, antibiotics as needed, steroids as needed, nutritional support, respiratory muscle training, and respiratory/cardiac rehabilitation, should be added. All of these interventions will play an additive role in improving the client's quality of life and reducing impending frailty. Thus, pulmonary rehabilitation is a very broad group of therapies that both the American Thoracic Society and European Respiratory Society call a *"comprehensive intervention and based on a thorough patient assessment followed by patient tailored therapies that include, but are not limited to exercise training, education and behavior change, designed to improve the physical and psychological condition of people with chronic respiratory disease and to promote the long-term adherence to health enhancing behaviors."*[31]

There is a global initiative for COPD treatment that suggests a rehabilitation program should be included in the management of clients with COPD.[32] Because frailty occurs in one quarter of clients with COPD, these clients may benefit greatly from pulmonary rehabilitation along with other frailty interventions. Studies have been done on frail individuals who completed pulmonary and or cardiac rehabilitation. Those individuals encountered reduced dyspnea (shortness of breath), improved exercise ability and physical activity levels, and sixty-one percent of those individuals no longer met the criteria for frailty.

Three screening questions for frailty in some of the frailty scoring systems include daily fatigue, an inability to walk one block, and the inability to climb one flight of stairs. All three factors could be improved with pulmonary rehabilitation in those clients with COPD with targeted activity prescriptions and optimization of medications for the respiratory condition present. The resistance and activity components of walking one block or climbing one flight of stairs

---

31 https://www.atsjournals.org/doi/10.1164/rccm.201309-1634ST

32 https://www.atsjournals.org/doi/10.1164/rccm.201309-1634ST

can be improved in the short, medium, and ultimately long-term with activity programs and long-term maintenance of activity. Frailty with chronic lung disease is *not* a contraindication to pulmonary rehabilitation programs. In fact, these clients may benefit the most from this type of program, which can be done in an institutionalized setting as a group, in an outpatient setting as a group, or in individual home pulmonary rehabilitation (where home care services provide this support). The home programs require a motivated client who is receptive to significant education sessions and instruction for various exercises. These include but are not limited to learning about helpful or efficient breathing techniques. Again, this chapter will elaborate what individual clients and families can do, especially if access to these programs or primary care is limited or non existent.

In the medical literature, clients who have an increase in their chronic CO_2 levels (hypercapnia) due to COPD have also been studied, and hypercapnia is *not a contraindication* to pulmonary rehabilitation. In fact, significant benefit has been seen in these individuals. The only clients who should **not** be initiating a respiratory rehabilitation or cardio exercise program, are those individuals who are at increased cardiac risk during exercise. Some of these conditions include uncontrolled ischemic cardiac disease (chest pain or angina), decompensated congestive heart failure (fluid build up in the lungs or body), profound pulmonary hypertension (high blood pressure in the lung vessels noted on echocardiogram), uncontrolled systemic hypertension (BP usually greater than 180/100 at rest), and those clients with known exercised-induced palpitations or arrhythmias. Sometimes, adjustments to the activity programs may need to be made when clients have certain conditions or obstacles that prevent them from participating in programs. These conditions could include severe arthritis, neurologic impairment with overt neurologic deficits (stroke causing paralysis or severe weakness of one or more of the limbs), or inability to follow commands as we see in cognitive impairment or dementia. There may also be other logistical or psychosocial issues, such as an inability to get transportation to the program.

In an ideal world, every participant who is thinking about an exercise program for their lungs should have a pulmonary assessment, which would include a history and physical examination, medication review, pulmonary function testing, an assessment of overall exercise tolerance either with six-minute walking oximetry or a plain cardiac stress test, and comprehensive review of any other illness or conditions (cardiac, musculoskeletal, and neurologic disease). Any deviations from normal in any of the above assessments, will require adjustments to the basic rehabilitation program. Again, individualization of any exercise regimen that will be sustained, is key for the patient to improve fitness and functionality. The inability to follow commands and instructions should trigger a screen for cognitive impairment, impaired hearing or vision, language barriers and other psychosocial factors.

The pulmonary function tests look at spirometry levels (how much air can one blowout in zero to six seconds) and the diffusing capacity CO (carbon monoxide), which tells clinicians if there is any significant impairment of oxygen getting from the lungs (breathing) and going into the systemic circulation (diffusion and circulation) and an overall exercise/functional capacity.[33]

You can use the Internet to search for "pulmonary rehabilitation programs near me" and will often get a local or provincial site or association to contact. If there is a local program available and if you've been diagnosed with COPD, your medications have been adjusted and stabilized, and you haven't recently been admitted to hospital for COPD exacerbation or pneumonia, you should contact your primary care provider or lung specialist to see if one of these programs would be beneficial for you.

In my opinion, clients should be referred to a pulmonary rehab program at least once after diagnosis to learn the basics of respiratory education (anatomy and physiology), breathing techniques, proper use of medications and exercise plans. However, many of us live in regions

---

33 "Lung Function Tests," American Lung Association, accessed August 23, 2022, https://www.lung.org/lung-health-diseases/lung-procedures-and-tests/lung-function-tests.

of the country where we don't have easy access to such programs.[34] The details in this chapter are targeted at those individuals.

If possible, I recommend the purchase of a pulse oximeter,[35] which is a small finger clip monitor that monitors your heart rate and oxygen saturations through your fingertip at rest and with exertion. These can easily be ordered online by a family member or purchased through large retailers or other electronics stores.

One of the simple screens you can do for determining your baseline fitness level is to do a six-minute walk test. What you're looking for is the total distance you can walk in six minutes, oxygen saturations during the walk, and symptoms of shortness of breath or chest pain during that walk. Formal completed pulmonary rehabilitation programs have shown that the average improvement in the six-minute walk was about 107 metres of improved mobility. An increase of thirty-five metres or more is considered significant. Of course, you would only do this initial assessment when you're feeling at your baseline and haven't recently been unwell with a viral or bacterial upper or lower respiratory tract infection, noticed a change in the colour or amount of sputum production, experienced new onset of coughing up blood, or have been recently hospitalized.

The goal would be to have a program to do, two to five days a week that would include a progressive walking regimen, depending on your baseline activity tolerance. This might mean walking in the mall in the winter time, walking outdoors with a "workout buddy," or going to a seniors' water fitness class. Clinicians would like clients with chronic lung disease to do a minimum of at least eight to twelve weeks of a home-based program, with the ultimate goal of doing these exercises as long as possible to *maintain fitness levels*. You can use the Dr. Karen's Perceived Exertion scale listed in Chapter 4. I would advocate that clients have a perceived exertion scale in the 3–5 range for several weeks before attempting to do a little more exertion

---

34 "Pulmonary Rehabilitation," Canadian Lung Association, accessed August 23, 2022, https://www.lung.ca/research/pulmonary-rehabilitation.

35 "Pulse Oximetry," Yale Medicine, accessed August 23, 2022, https://www.yalemedicine.org/conditions/pulse-oximetry.

(6–7 range). Exercise would need to be interrupted immediately if clients develop any symptoms such as light-headedness, fainting, palpitations, rapid heart rate, low blood pressure, chest pain, or your pulse oximeter showing that your pulse oximetry is persistently under eighty-eight percent.

While formal pulmonary rehabilitation programs have many components and include many team members, with a high quality of respiratory education, these programs are not always available to every client with chronic lung disease. These programs focus on encouraging exercise training and the promotion of healthy behaviours such as tobacco cessation, nutrition, proper medication and bronchodilator use (including compliance) in the home. As with any chronic illness, teaching clients the concepts of self management and action plans for when symptoms flare, are also key learning points that may help to keep these clients out of hospital. Psychological support is also available in many programs.

If these programs are not available, I do think that individuals attempting a home program, need to find a suitable friend, spouse, home care worker, coach, respiratory therapist, psychologist, physiotherapist, occupational therapist, or community mental health worker to work with if the client is unsure if the individual can do this alone. The Canadian Lung Association has a great website to assist in your lung education and treatment goals. There are even detailed instructions on how to use your prescribed inhalers. If you're a smoker or have been diagnosed with COPD, it's *never* too early to seek out advice from a reputable community organization such as this one (lung.ca).

There are many exercise limitations with chronic lung disease that are beyond the scope of this discussion, but these physiological limitations include ventilatory and gas transfer abnormalities, pulmonary vascular impairments and overall cardiac dysfunction. There can also be skeletal muscle (arms/legs) dysfunction and illnesses that can interfere with adequate generation of activity. While there may be many impairments to exercise, if successful reconditioning and muscle strength improves, AND these changes make you feel better, less frail, and more energetic, why wouldn't you try?

My suggestion for initiating home endurance training for COPD clients is to start with using a similar exercise program to those patients with congestive heart failure, in which you'll slowly try to achieve thirty minutes of exercise at seventy percent of your age-predicted maximum, five times a week (BASIC EXERCISE PLAN #2)

This workload can also be achieved by using stationary bicycles, minibikes, treadmills, and elliptical trainers. Other methods of activity can include walking, swimming, attending aqua fit sessions, climbing stairs, or dancing to get your heart rate up to that range. On the first day, after a five-minute warmup and followed by a five-minute cool down, do whatever small amount of exercise makes you feel that you're working on Karen's Exertion Scale at 3–4 (see Chapter 4). After that initial episode, the "cardio" portion should be increased by one minute every day that you attempt the training sessions. If you're too short of breath, you can scale back the intensity of activity, the time or even changing activities. I would like to see an initial attempt at an exercise program for at least four weeks before giving up. The ultimate goal, is to get individuals doing some activities, five to seven days a week, within your breathing capabilities (ideally 150 minutes per week).

As with all clients, doing lower extremity exercises if one has chronic lung disease, is necessary for all of us. We rely on our leg strength to get us in and out of bed, for sitting and standing from the toilet, moving from chair to chair and many other basic activities of daily living. COPD can result in malnutrition due to the increased work of breathing which can worsen weakness as well. In order to improve the lower extremity fitness, strength, endurance, and flexibility, everyone with or without COPD needs to improve the overall strength and functionality of those leg muscles.

Clients with COPD might not achieve the same muscle building and strength building goals, if the work of breathing at rest is excessive or end stage. If this is the case, individuals should continue to do ANY activities that are within the comfortable breathing limits of the disease process. Lower leg exercises may need to be adjusted for individual's specific overall status. Clinicians know that resistance training may improve an individual's work of breathing subjectively, but the absolute change in pulmonary function tests likely will not change. Thus, exercise programs improve a client's symptoms and that is definitely, worth the effort.

As with leg training, upper extremity exercise is also important, as almost all of our everyday tasks require the use of arms, forearms, wrists, elbows, and shoulders. The next chapter will detail how to embark on leg and arm exercise training, and those clients with chronic lung disease should start at a low level and slowly increase repetitions up to a tolerable level as breathing or energy permit.

If you want to know how bad your COPD is, there are prediction scores that give estimates of overall survival. For clinicians, these are available from numerous medical calculator websites. For understanding where an individual's symptoms are at, the mMRC dyspnea scale (modified Medical Research Council) quantifies inability to function based on breathlessness.[36]

Dyspnea with only strenuous exercise	0	definitely start a program
Dyspnea when hurrying or walking up a slight hill	+1	start a more advanced activity program and reduce intensity if needed
Walks slower than people of same age because of dyspnea OR stops for breath when walking at own pace	+2	start a lower level activity program but reduce intensity if needed
Stops for breath after walking ninety-one metres	+3	range of motion, stretching, limited walking, brain and balance exercises
Too dyspneic to leave house or breathless with dressing	+4	bed, chair, balance, and brain exercises

As a clinician, I would advise that mMRC scores of 0, +1 or +2 can start the activity programs as suggested in this book. For those individuals with mMRC scores of +3 or +4, I would advise only brain, balance, and very limited resistance exercises to maintain mobility with activities of daily living. Other cardio regimens should be undertaken in these severely symptomatic individuals, only as part of a comprehensive and *supervised* formal pulmonary rehabilitation program.

---

36 https://www.pcrs-uk.org

The following chapter will detail how to improve muscle strength with resistance training, and in Chapter 7, I will discuss balance training exercise that would be appropriate for anyone with or without chronic lung disease.

Pulmonary rehabilitation education focuses on breathing retraining; short, shallow breaths are not very efficient. Yoga and pursed lip breathing have led to increasing breathing volume and oxygen saturation and a reduction in the feeling of being short of breath. Diaphragmatic breathing (using the large chest muscle that separates the chest cavity from the abdominal cavity), seems to increase the tidal volume through focusing on diaphragmatic descent. While the medical studies of diaphragmatic breathing show different outcomes, anytime you can decrease your overall respiratory rate and prolong the time it takes for you to expire the air from your lungs, it will help with COPD, hyperinflation, and the sensation of being short of breath.

A formal pulmonary rehabilitation program would provide educational components including normal anatomy and physiology of the lung, and abnormal/pathophysiology of the lung in COPD. You would also learn about breathing training, energy conservation, medications, other self-management skills, indications for oxygen therapy, and avoiding stressful abnormal environments (hot humid days, forest fire smoke, pollution). In advanced academic or large urban programs, access to a respiratory therapist or other allied health professional, will also assist with teaching respiratory and chest physiotherapy techniques, symptom management and end-of-life planning. Of the above topics I briefly mentioned in this paragraph, the most exceptional service is always provided by a formal respiratory rehabilitation program taught by respiratory therapists or chronic disease management nurses/allied health educators. [37] That being said, with our current limitations in primary care, any educational component that focuses on any of the topics will all help prepare you for self management of your chronic medical condition.

One of the important parts of general health preservation is vaccinations. Seasonal influenza vaccination, pneumococcal vaccination,

---

37 https://www.technologyforliving.org/provincial-respiratory-outreach-program-prop/

COVID-19 vaccination, and even possibly Haemophilus influenza B vaccination and shingles vaccination need to be considered. Individuals need to reach out to your primary care provider or lung specialist or public health unit to review your vaccination history. A discussion about the benefits and risks of receiving any or all of the vaccinations listed, or upcoming new vaccination strategies, is required with your health-care team or public health department.

Medication adherence with prescribed oral and inhaled medications is critical to keeping you out of hospital. If there are any physical limitations to you using your puffer correctly, liaise with your pharmacist, community respiratory therapist, and/or primary care provider for some respiratory education on proper puffer use. Usually, antibiotics are needed for bacterial infections and sometimes COPD exacerbations. Occasionally, you might be prescribed an indefinite long-term antibiotic to prevent exacerbations, as there are some anti-inflammatory effects. A drug called azithromycin is often used in this regard, which can be given as a low-dose daily or three times per week for up to one year. Your lung specialist is the best physician to discuss this strategy with if you find yourself repeatedly being hospitalized for your COPD.

Another important lung health preservation strategy is screening for sleep apnea and lung cancer. If you have been an extensive smoker in the past, then a self referral program for lung cancer screening is available in many areas now. This is done by getting a low dose CT thorax to rule out lung cancer.

Sleep apnea is incredibly common and leads to further cardio-respiratory disease and premature death if not treated. A screening questionnaire that you can do at home and drop off at a neighborhood sleep clinic/vendor may be required. If partners notice that clients snore and stop breathing while sleeping, this needs an urgent assessment through your primary care provider, local sleep apnea/oxygen depot, respiratory services clinic, or sleep specialist.

Please review the Canadian Lung association website for proper instructions on using your puffers.

Below is a proposed basic exercise regimen for clients with respiratory disease that is not too severe.

BASIC EXERCISE PRESCRIPTION FOR COPD PATIENTS (mMRC scale 0, +1, +2):

WEEK	BED/BRAIN EXERCISES	ROM/BALANCE/ BREATHING	BASIC CARDIO #2	PROGRESSION
1	START WEEK 1	--	--	--
2	CONTINUE	START WEEK 2	--	--
3	CONTINUE	CONTINUE	START WEEK 3	SEE BASIC CARDIO #2 FOR GRID
4	CONTINUE	CONTINUE	CONTINUE	PROGRESS AS PER BASIC CARDIO #2
5	CONTINUE	CONTINUE	CONTINUE	PROGRESS AS PER BASIC CARDIO #2
6	CONTINUE	CONTINUE	CONTINUE	PROGRESS AS PER BASIC CARDIO #2
7–8	CONTINUE	CONTINUE	CONTINUE	PROGRESS AS PER BASIC CARDIO #2
9–10	CONTINUE	CONTINUE	CONTINUE	PROGRESS AS PER BASIC CARDIO #2
11+	CONTINUE	CONTINUE	CONTINUE	PROGRESS AS PER BASIC CARDIO #2

Add in weight training after week 8. See Chapter 7 for details.

CHAPTER SUMMARY

In this chapter, I have discussed the components and benefits of pulmonary rehab programs. Outside of large centres, there is a paucity of formal programs. Review with your primary care provider, clinic nurse, respirologist, pharmacist, or community respiratory therapist how to take your puffers and how to do breathing exercises.

If you do not have access to primary care or lung specialists, and you have a known diagnosis of COPD or have symptoms suggestive of COPD, here are some guidelines to access care and initiate your own program:

1. Engage a family member to help you advocate for primary care
    a. Contact the lung association or local community resources for lung care if available
    b. This might mean trying to get into a walk-in clinic, an urgent primary care centre and/or getting on a registry or waiting list to get a primary care provider
    c. Ask around, look on the Internet, contact your MLAs office and or government website
    d. Progressive symptoms and impaired function require a hospital assessment (ER or admission)
    e. When you have the attention of a care provider, review your symptoms as listed in this Chapter and keep a journal of your symptoms and mMRC score
        i. Ask the provider for a referral to lung specialist (especially if you don't have access to primary care)
        ii. Ask for a respiratory therapist to do some teaching while in the health care system or as an outpatient referral
        iii. Ask the nurse, respiratory therapist, or community pharmacist for a lesson on how to use your prescribed puffers correctly
        iv. Ask the discharging clinician for a "COPD ACTION PLAN" for education when to increase puffers, add other medications and when to return to the hospital
2. Get your vaccinations up to date by contacting your local public health unit
3. Once you are stable on current medications for your COPD, ask for a formal pulmonary function test to be arranged so that you know your FEV1 – with any clinician visit
4. When at your baseline, purchase a pulse oximeter to get to know your resting and activity related oxygen saturation levels and heart rates

a. Engage a family member to help you do a six-minute walk test
    i. Track BP and heart rate
    ii. Track oximetry
    iii. Track symptoms
    iv. Track length of walk achieved in the six minutes
b. This is your current baseline
c. With your family member, friend, or coach present
    i. Start your activity program as listed in this chapter if your mMRC score is 0, 1 or 2
d. Do not attempt exercising on your own (cardio or resistance) if your mMRC score is 3 or 4.
    i. You can still participate in the brain, balance, bed, and range of motion exercises listed in the next chapter
    ii. At the next interaction with the health care system – ask for a referral to a formal pulmonary rehabilitation program when your symptoms are back to YOUR baseline

Everyone with COPD would benefit from at least one two-week community pulmonary rehabilitation program for learning basic lung anatomy and physiology and training exercises to improve quality of life.

Community respiratory therapists are instrumental in teaching the concepts of breathing exercises, puffer utilization, and energy conservation. As COPD and frailty often co exist, even the most severely frail COPD clients will benefit from a progressive pulmonary rehabilitation.

CHAPTER 6:
ESSENTIALS OF LOW RESISTANCE WEIGHT TRAINING

There is no elevator to success, each one of us has to take the stairs.
—Zig Ziglar[38]

In the last two chapters, I focused on specific cardiac and pulmonary rehabilitation principles. In this chapter, I will focus on the benefits of using resistance training in order to reduce the progression of, or diminish, frailty and weakness. In the medical literature, there has been meta-analyses done looking at different exercise regimens in frailty. There is low to moderate evidence that appropriate cardio exercise and low-level weight/resistance training is beneficial in any age group, including pre-frail and frail clients.

As a physician, my recommendation for weight training is quite simple. First and foremost, joints and muscles must have adequate range of motion before any resistance is added. Any adult needs to start any activity program by first moving the major joints and muscle groups, in the normal ranges of motion. This includes full range of motion (without strain!) of the neck and spine, arms, elbows, shoulders, wrists, hips, knees, and ankles. Range of motion itself is a dedicated warm up for most activities but as adults, we need to remind ourselves to do these activities purposefully and daily. A regimen of doing upper limbs and spine on even days alternating with lower limbs and core/abdominal muscles on odd days is a good start. The range of motion consists of 8-12 repetitions for each range of motion exercise for each joint/muscle group, on each side of the body. This can be repeated as needed for flexibility throughout the day. This requires at least two weeks of dedicated range of motion practice BEFORE any resistance can be added to the regimen.

---

38 Inspirational quote; Zig Ziglar June 18, 2019

I also favour exercises such as yoga, Tai Chi, and lap swimming to facilitate movement of many muscle groups at once. Tai Chi and yoga both can improve balance and flexibility as well, but not every individual has access to those activities in many communities. In the past, I have downloaded beginner Tai Chi from YouTube videos and practised in the privacy of my back yard. If one does not have access to programs that offer these services, they can use some of the wellness channels on TV for instructions as well.

If you have resistance tubing or small weights such as 1- or 2-pound dumbbells, then after the first two weeks you can add in exercises such as biceps curls and triceps extensions. Many individuals feel comfortable in starting these sort of low resistance activities without supervision or ask family or friends for a quick lesson on the weight training basics.

However, many people feel unsure about starting these on their own and seek out either an exercise trainer, private physiotherapist, kinesiologist, or they buy a membership to a gym to learn proper exercise technique. These lessons improve the individuals comfort level in starting a new regimen. The goal of obtaining this sort of instruction would be to facilitate strength training with less concerns about injuries due to improper technique. These facilitators also instruct on the slow progression of activities to ensure the client is not moving through the exercise program too quickly or with bad form.

Injuries are possible at any time and increase with advancing age and lack of conditioning. Proper technique and a slowly progressive program are the keys to avoiding injuries. Individuals should be reminded to participate in activity programs only when they are feeling well and at their baseline, before embarking on light resistance training exercises and cardio regimens.

If you are feeling unwell, it is not the time to push your body. If you have an illness that lasts more than twenty-four hours, you must allow your body forty-eight hours to get back to its baseline before pursuing cardio regimens or weight training programs. Once you do start back on your program, you should only be doing twenty-five to fifty percent of the usual workload the first day and increase that workload by twenty-five percent daily until your back at your usual baseline. If you are hospitalized or ill for more than two weeks, you essentially have to start your cardio and resistance regimens from the beginning, as if you were starting all over again. Deconditioning in hospital can happen to even the most elite athlete, depending upon the illness.

If clients, family members, or health care providers need further input, the article by Fragal et al can provide further information.[39]

This is an extensive and thorough document that looks at all the evidence-based literature and goes into quite a bit of detail regarding resistance training for older adults. There are also 663 referenced articles in this paper if clients, health care providers, or their families wish to seek out additional data.

The general principles of resistance training guidelines for adults with frailty include:

Frequency: Perform two to three times per week

Number of sets/repetitions: work up to three sets of eight to twelve repetitions

Definition of 1 RM: 1RM is the maximum amount of weight that one can successfully (with proper form) do in one attempt.

Intensity #1: intensity that starts at 20 percent of 1RM for the first week and increases by 20 percent each week until progressing to 80 percent of 1RM.

Intensity #2: Exercises at high speed of motion and lower intensity (i.e., 30–60 percent of 1RM) will induce marked improvements in the functional task performance

The concept of functional training includes exercises in which daily activities are simulated, such as the sit-to-stand exercise. Other

---

39 RESISTANCE TRAINING FOR OLDER ADULTS: POSITION STATEMENT FORM THE NATIONAL STRENGTH AND CONDITIONING ASSOCIATION; Fragala et al. Journal of Strength and Conditioning Research: August 2019-Volume 33-Issue 8-p 2019-2052.

examples include squatting down to pick up something on the floor and doing this repeatedly as an exercise or lifting one's buttocks off the chair with arms only and holding the pose for a few seconds before lowering the buttocks back down into the chair. This too can be repeated.

When does an individual with frailty start with resistance training?

Once range of motion of the joints has been mastered for at least two weeks, then functional training can be initiated at any point thereafter. After one week of functional training, the individual can start with adding resistance tubing or small weights (1-2 lbs) and start upper arm biceps and triceps exercises on even days. On odd days, straight leg raises, bent leg raises can be done in the seated position in a chair. Squats at the kitchen sink can be added as tolerated to this regimen.

What should be done first – resistance training or cardio regimens??

Ideally, low level cardio (Basic regimen #2 and range of motion can be initiated at the same time along with balance and brain training—see chapter 7. Functional exercises can be initiated starting week 3 and low-level resistance training can be started on week 4.

Remember from Chapter 4, basic cardio regimen #2 starts with walking and progression to walking with changes in speed (walking like you're late for school), incline (doing hills), treadmill walking (in which you can vary the speed and incline of the treadmill), step-ups (using a stable step-up bench or the bottom stair of a flight of stairs with a handrail to hang onto for balance/safety), progressive stair climbing, basement, local arena, or other stairs in the community, and stationary biking with mini bike or recumbent bike.

Start at five to ten minutes for one of these activities per day and then add one to two minutes to the time in the activity every 1-3 activity sessions. Then, eventually progress to fifteen to thirty minutes of the chosen activity or activities, most days of the week. Taking one or two rest days per week is encouraged!

Using Karen's Exertion Scale in Chapter 4, the first week should be at stage 2–3, the second week at 4–5, and the third week at 6–7, with a goal of exertion scale 7–8 as a long-term goal.

There may be exercise modifications required for some conditions and consider these next statements as suggestions to consider for the following conditions.

Frailty (FRAIL SCORE 4-5)

Consider doing bed exercises for the first two to three weeks. Remember to start at a lower resistance, progress more slowly, and limit end point to the start of muscle fatigue (I am tired but I can still do a little, but I am not hurting).

Remember, the overall goal for NONFRAIL individuals is to start at 8–12 reps at 20 percent of 1RM and progress to 80 percent of 1RM. The frail client can start and progress at much lower and slower levels. In this case, it is more important to do what one can and progress if one can, rather that strict goals of progressing at a certain rate.

Mobility Limitations

This would include symptoms such as dizziness, BP drops with standing, peripheral neuropathy, stroke with balance or other mobility deficits, visual impairment, use of walking aids

Consider exercises in seated position. If joining a gym is possible, asking for a trainer to teach the client proper technique on the weight machines, may be more beneficial to the client. Use resistance tubing rather than free weights if there is a risk of dropping the weights and injuring oneself.

Mild Cognitive Impairment

In these cases, the family member or trainer needs to select simple, one step exercises. These clients will require extra instruction and demonstration, possibly at every exercise session. I would recommend a workout buddy/chaperone/accountability partner in this situation.

Diabetes

Please monitor your blood glucose levels before and after training. Do not exercise without having fuel to burn, by eating one to two hours ahead of planned exercise session. Sometimes, I do not take my diabetic medications until after I have done my work out to ensure I am not going too low when I am walking, miles away from home. You will need to discuss this with your diabetic education team or primary care provider. I also ensure I have access to high glucose content, short acting carbohydrates on hand if I do experience any symptoms of hypoglycemia. This was a greater concern when I was on insulin as part of my diabetic regimen and is less of a concern for me now.

Remember, that long standing diabetics may have undiagnosed cardiovascular disease, nerve disease, kidney disease, eye disease, and neuropathies, which may impose mobility or safety limitations, before embarking upon an unsupervised exercise program. It is always best to have an exercise "buddy," exercise in locations with cell phone signal and have a functioning cell phone on hand in the event of any unforeseen events.

Osteoporosis

If you have osteoporosis, please begin at a lower intensity for resistance training after the two weeks of range of motion activities. One can attempt the balance training, but at all costs, prevent falls whenever possible. Focus on form and technique and use caution with bending and twisting. Include postural exercises such as spinal extension but never force the body to do more than what is comfortable. If you have joint pain or limited range of motion (arthritis), consider the use of machines to avoid the joints or muscles "giving out" when using free weights. There is some need to work through a minimal amount of limb pain to allow for training through the "pain free" range of motion and then progress to attain a noticeable improvement. Pre-treatment with an anti-inflammatory medication (if prescribed, and one has no history of hypertension, peptic ulcer disease, chronic kidney disease, congestive heart failure or other known contraindications) or Tylenol may assist in getting through you workout.

Poor vision, equilibrium, and balance issues (falling), low-back pain, and dropping weight

Please consider using weight machines (as opposed to free weights) once instructions have been received as these may be safer in the long run.

Remember, if you are doing cardio exercise regimen #1, you can do your light weight resistance training to the same degree of exertion, Karen Exertion Scale (5–8). However, if you're on the gentle cardio exercise regimen #2, then your resistance training also needs to be a lower level, with an exertion score of (3–6).

These are my basic guidelines that provide a starting point, to get the client thinking about and progressing with a program. All programs will eventually need to be individualized for each client scenario. If you need assistance with an exercise program for you, consider other sources to review, and seek out coaches, trainers, physiotherapists, or kinesiologists as required.[40] [41] [42] [43]

I don't always suggest tracking with a Fitbit or Apple watch unless the client already has those items. The heart rate assessment with exercise programs may be helpful for individuals keen on reviewing these and other parameters in response to exercise. Over the years, I've

---

40 Accessed August 23, 2022, https://loveyourage.ca/.

41 "Could You Use an Exercise Prescription?" Heart&Stroke, accessed August 23, 2022, https://www.heartandstroke.ca/articles/could-you-use-an-exercise-prescription.

42 "Diabetes Care Providers Spring into Action," Acadia University, April 25, 2012, https://www2.acadiau.ca/home/news-reader-page/diabetes-care-providers-spring-into-action.html.

43 Accessed August 23, 2022, https://guidelines.diabetes.ca/docs/resources/diabetes-and-physical-activity-your-exercise-prescription.pdf.

found that perceived exertion scales give clients an idea of their target heart rate when they're working out. Light to somewhat hard (3–6) is for patients who have frailty, COPD, heart disease or congestive heart failure, and hard to very hard (6–8) is for most of the other clients.

CHAPTER SUMMARY

Once you've been doing bed, balance, and brain activities, you can move on to range of motion and then light resistance weight training, along with a low-level cardio regimen (Basic #2). All activities need to be adjusted for the individual. There may be some exercise that one just can't do. Don't fret; any activity is better than none. Let your body guide you, and don't feel you need to keep the same intensity level as a workout partner or spouse. Progress at your own pace, and if you truly can't progress, then liaise with your health-care team to see if there is any underlying illness that needs to be addressed.

CHAPTER 7:
BALANCE AND BRAIN TRAINING FOR ADULTS OF ALL AGES

Life is like riding a bicycle … To keep your balance … you must keep moving. —Albert Einstein

In the last chapter, I spoke primarily of low resistance weight training exercises. These alone, will help with increasing muscle strength as long as there are no underlying conditions that limit muscle strength training. I feel that strength in large muscle groups is one of the keys to having CONFIDENCE to initiate or continue with an activity program. The other key component for confidence to participate is a sense of good balance. In this chapter, I will speak about self care balance exercises and programs that most adults can initiate on their own.

In Canadian medical school training, we rarely talk about balance training for older adults. Yet in other parts of the world, yoga, meditation, Tai Chi, and other exercises have been well known to improve balance, flexibility, stamina, and calmness. As we age, balance loss occurs often in situations when one's attention is divided. Balance control, is a complicated process involving many of the body systems that need to coordinate with one another and regulate the many systems all at once. In order to exercise and train those integrated systems, individuals need to do dedicated and progressive balance training exercises.

Balance training can include many exercises, such as line walking, tandem foot standing, standing on one leg, heel-toe walking, stepping practice, and weight transfers from one leg to the other.

Once basic balance exercises have been mastered, I also suggest the addition of other tasks such as additional physical and mental tasks.

Progression may include a gradual increase in the volume, intensity, and complexity of the exercises. In addition to complexity of exercises, adding in stimuli like counting to ten, reciting the alphabet, singing a song, opening and then closing eyes, adding in arm movements while balancing on one leg or a combination of these tasks as one progresses, can assist in balance improvements. Ultimately, the goal of improved balance is fall-prevention. Further information for balance training is widely available but I have included a reference below.[44]

In this study by Halverson et al, they illustrate how a group of clients were instructed on balance-demanding exercises, specific to the various components of balance control and situations in daily life. These were performed while sitting, standing, and walking at three different levels of progression (basic, moderate, and advanced) of increasing difficulty and complexity. This was a group training program for forty-five minutes, three times per week, for twelve weeks. The participants numbered from six to ten in each group, with two to three physiotherapists present for safety measures.

In this program, they found that the balance training program strength and self-sufficiency and balance control, leading to improved fall related self-sufficiency, reduce fear of falling, increased walking speed, and improved physical function. Clients in the programs found their program motivating, valuable, fun, and enjoyable, which was reflected in a high attendance rate. These kinds of programs also provide an opportunity for social prescribing and interactions for those seniors who are socially isolated.[45]

At any point, anyone can seek out such a program, and I advise clients to look at the local chapters of CARP (Canadian Association of Retired Persons) or other resources, but I will provide you with some simple balance exercises one can do at home.

We need good balance to do just about everything, including walking, getting out of bed, getting out of a chair, and leaning over to tie up our shoelaces. Being strong and steady and sometimes flexible are all required to make those things happen. While some yoga poses can be very challenging, if you're accustomed to doing yoga,

---

44 "Taking Balance Training for Older Adults One Step Further: The Rationale for and a Description of a Proven Balance Training Programme," National Library of Medicine, September 8, 2014, https://pubmed.ncbi.nlm.nih.gov/25200877/.

45 Bennell and Hinman.

I'd recommend continue doing yoga, Tai Chi, or Pilates. If you don't already have a balance program, then some of these exercises can be incorporated into your daily routine.

Each morning while waiting for my coffee to brew, I stand on one leg, and I'm either raising the other leg to the side or behind me. I stand at the kitchen counter and have access to grasp the sink/counter if my balance starts to falter. I do this on each side ten to fifteen times. I move on to trying to stand on one leg and putting the heel of my other leg just above my knee (yoga tree pose) on my inner thigh, and I count how long I can stay in this position without losing balance. I aim for an additional second of balance every day I do this. Again, I'm by myself but I'm near the counter if my balance starts to fail. Safety is *always* one's first priority.

I then walk ten steps on my toes to the fridge to get my coffee cream, and I walk back on my heels to put the cream in my coffee. I do that with every coffee refill. I also balance on one leg and lift my entire body weight with my toes on that leg, bringing my heel up and down for ten to fifteen repetitions. And I repeat on the other side. Finally, I stand with feet together in front of the sink, with my arms stretched out to the side. I close my eyes and alternate touching my index finger to my nose five times on each hand.

While these are simple things one can do that take only a few minutes a day while you're waiting for your coffee to finish brewing, other options are to join a yoga or Tai Chi class, or use equipment like a Bosu ball, which has an inflatable dome on top of a circular platform on which you can balance. I would recommend the Bosu ball exercises only under supervision with a spotter/chaperone to assist in the first few weeks.

As the weeks go by, my goal is to hold the position for a longer amount of time, adding a different movement or breathing activity to the activities, such as singing a song or reciting the alphabet, or closing my eyes for periods of time. No balance exercise regimen is complete without some core abdominal strength training. For this task, I tend to use planks. Core strengthening exercise are ideal but not always tolerated in every age group.

When I'm at work, I often do the balance and some of the resistance training while on a break or outside enjoying the weather.

You can also research various websites to review illustrations of how to do many balance activities.[46]

As with all of the recommendations in this book, exercises should be performed with proper form and technique, which should be established with a qualified family member or instructor before exercise progression occurs and keep proper form and technique in mind, during progression of these activity programs.

CAUTION: When engaging in balance exercises and basic range of motion activities, have something to hang on to, and ideally practise when someone can be with you. These exercises below can be done at any fitness level and with most conditions.

Balance Program A – Adding in Balance to range of motion (ROM) weeks at the same time.

Week	Range of Motion: Arms	Range of Motion: Legs, Knees, Ankles	Balance Exercises	Yoga or Tai chi or Pilates	Number of Repetitions Per Day	Goals for Progression
1	5–10 repetitions for each muscle group	5–10 repetitions for each muscle group	5–10	As desired/tolerated	1–2	Slowly increase balance time
2	5–10 repetitions for each muscle group	5–10 repetitions for each muscle group	8–12	As desired/tolerated	2–3	Slowly increase time with balancing exercises as tolerated
3	5–10 repetitions for each muscle group	5–10 repetitions for each muscle group	8–12	As desired/tolerated	3	ROM still essential but if moving to weight training regimens, can limit ROM to one rep and then move on to resistance training**

---

46 "14 Exercises for Seniors to Improve Strength and Balance," Lifeline, accessed August 24, 2022, https://www.lifeline.ca/en/resources/14-exercises-for-seniors-to-improve-strength-and-balance/.

Week	Range of Motion: Arms	Range of Motion: Legs, Knees, Ankles	Balance Exercises	Yoga or Tai chi or Pilates	Number of Repetitions Per Day	Goals for Progression
4	5–10 repetitions for each muscle group	5–10 repetitions for each muscle group	8–12	As desired/tolerated	3**	ROM still essential but if moving to weight training regimens, can limit ROM to one rep and then move on to resistance training**
5–8	5–10 repetitions for each muscle group	5–10 repetitions for each muscle group	8–12	As desired/tolerated	3**	ROM still essential but if moving to weight training regimens, can limit ROM to one rep and then move on to resistance training**
9–12	5–10 repetitions for each muscle group	5–10 repetitions for each muscle group	8–12	As desired/tolerated	3**	ROM still essential but if moving to weight training regimens, can limit ROM to one rep and then move on to resistance training**
13+	5–10 repetitions for each muscle group	5–10 repetitions for each muscle group	8–12	As desired/tolerated	3**	ROM still essential but if moving to weight training regimens, can limit ROM to one rep and then move on to resistance training**

I incorporate balance and brain training in one chapter as some of the balance tasks, are a form of brain training as well. Having both adequate balance and cognitive function empowers seniors to keep living a safe life, in their own home. If balance and brain training can not be improved with these activities, and the senior is not considered to be safe alone at home, then the individual needs to consider the concept of assistance in the home, relocation and/or downsizing.

I'd like to discuss the concept of "downsizing" or "smart-sizing" which is a term most seniors don't want to hear. When an individual's balance and cognitive fitness level make living alone in a large home unsafe, those individuals need to explore other living arrangements. What is the optimal size to live in as we age? As we get older, we tend to use only a very small amount of space. It is estimated by the "Engineers Toolbox" that many individuals can live in 100-400 sq ft.[47] This is likely some of the data that has piqued the interest in "tiny homes." For the older adult, this requirement to change living arrangements comes with some heavy psychological burden. Along with this concept of "downsizing," the psychological burden of possibly not being able to drive a car in the near future also is a heavy burden. There is anticipatory grieving for the perceived loss of independence and all the "stuff" that the homeowner may need to purge. This can be a challenging time for families, including my own.

My eighty-eight-year-old father is physically debilitated but cognitively intact. He can tell me more about current events than I know, and he has a fondness for watching old Western movies. Before he was physically limited, he was a superior carpenter and did a lot of work around his home before moving to an assisted living residence. He had to downsize tremendously, which meant all his carpentry tools were given away or sold. He was already mentally prepared to move to an assisted living residence before my mother passed away, which made his transition much easier. I would say to any family member anticipating having to go through these changes with your loved one soon, please be gentle when exploring these options. Your loved one may not be ready to discuss this inevitable process. This may also be a good time to explore if the activities in this book can help diminish or delay the need for relocation. While the suggestions in this book are hopefully going to decrease the need for relocation, the

---

47 http://online.wsj.com/article/SB10001424052702304708604577504672437027392.
   html

ability for families to openly discuss those options as soon as feasible does make sense. First of all, it gives the senior the option of trying to improve overall condition (I hope this book really does help!). Secondly, it allows the senior as much control in the process of timing and ultimate destination decision making, hopefully before an illness or hospitalization dictates otherwise. Much like teenagers and young adults believe they are invincible, most seniors don't really acknowledge that something devastating can happen to them in their own home, until it happens to a friend, family member, acquaintance, or celebrity. The sooner we openly discuss these concepts and possibilities with our loved ones, the easier it will be to accept and plan for this change when it becomes necessary. I always tell patients that they want to move when they're still able to enjoy the move and control what cherished items go with them. Having someone else do this for you because you've been hospitalized and are never going to be able to go home/ say goodbye to your favourite parts of the house and yard is not ideal.

Sometimes older adults are offended when family members bring up these possibilities. For those older adults reading this book, I guarantee that your loving family has initiated this conversation because they can see some concerning changes, deterioration or slowing down. If you fall, trip frequently (with or without injuries), look like you're barely able to manage your house or yard work, someone will inevitably mention downsizing and moving. It's important for the older adult to control the narrative at this point in your life. You don't want anyone making these decisions for you, so when the topic is broached, I urge you to listen carefully and start thinking about acceptable options for the future.

In my research, I do acknowledge that most adults need very little space to live as one ages. This is one of the big changes noted by older adults, if a move to a senior's residence, assisted living facility or personal (long-term) care home is anticipated. In addition to the change in living accommodation square footage, the cost is another challenging topic. Institutionalization is expensive! In contemplation of living well as we age, we need to keep our fitness and functionality along with our cognitive function at an acceptable level to survive by ourselves. When those things are no longer present, there will be an acceleration of that "last move" from you own home to likely your *final* place of residence. Every client needs supportive family and financial means to make those decisions. Our fitness and cognition, which would include how we think and solve problems, needs to be maintained for as long as possible. This next part of the chapter will discuss how our ability to think clearly and problem solve can improve with certain brain activities.

There are many ways to keep our brain active. It's important to treat underlying depression because the medications can make a world of difference to your outlook in life. Depression will be discussed later in the book, and even though you may not feel comfortable admitting to impaired mood, getting treated will likely improve your quality of life.

Avoiding alcohol is another way to keep your cognitive function intact. While quality of life may revolve around having an occasional glass of wine, each individual has to look at their own alcohol consumption and the pleasure, or lack thereof, they receive by drinking ethanol. If alcohol consumption is clearly part of your quality of life, you can reduce your intake or not. If you find there are more downsides to drinking alcohol, you may choose to abstain. Either way, this is your decision to make. If alcohol consumption is excessive, there are prescribed medications to assist you to quit drinking if you have a concern that ethanol consumption is excessive or causing harm. Please reach out to your primary care provider to discuss this further. Community supports are also available through a variety of programs.

There are *no* supplements that have been *proven* in the medical literature to improve cognition. My advice would be to not waste money on supplements but put it toward costs of future care or an exercise fund to do different activities on occasion. While there has been no proven benefit to over-the-counter health supplements, many clients still take them. As we age, our body metabolizes drugs less efficiently, and a lot of supplemental herbs and vitamins contribute to polypharmacy, which can impair your cognition further.

Your thinking may improve with regular medication reviews. Deprescribing may be offered by your primary care provider and occasionally, but a community pharmacist. In my opinion, medication reviews should be done every six to twenty-four months, depending on the complexity of your medication regimen and the availability of suitability trained team members to embark upon this task.

What can anyone do to promote brain health?

Our brain is a fantastic organ and scientists now know that the brain pathways are constantly updating and has the ability to change. This is a concept called "neuroplasticity" and the details are beyond the scope of this book. However, you CAN CHANGE the structural neuroplasticity by doing and learning new things.

Some specific brain exercises include:

- playing cards
- playing board games
- doing crossword puzzles/word search/sudoku
- learning a new language
- meditation
- practising gratitude
- socializing
- learning a new skill
- reading books
- writing hand-written cards or letters to family and friends
- learning computer skills
- emailing or texting friends and family
- listening to your favourite music or a new genre of music
- learning to play a musical instrument
- taking a class or a course
- teaching a class or course
- journaling your thoughts on a daily basis
- doing gardening and crafts
- watching certain TV shows that you like to follow
- cleaning your home
- paying attention to your budget and financial circumstances
- interacting with other generations

And of course, the benefit of exercise is improvement of blood flow to the entire body, including the brain. Social isolation should be avoided if possible, and activities such as square dancing or other dancing may also enhance one's brain function and socialization at the same time.

I tried to send my father watercolour pencil crayons, as I was an avid painter. He may have used them once, but he gets a lot more use from the several crossword puzzle and word search books I bought at the dollar store.

Other options include being artistic, practising mental math, or practising mathematics on paper. These all contribute to improving our brain activity. A simple start for anyone would be to review what you're grateful for everyday, document what you did for pleasure and for your brain health, and document whether you were kind to yourself/others. Start keeping a journal that includes these positive notes to reaffirm that there are many positives in your life, instead of focusing on what is negative in the world around you. This will help with making your brain change the way it processes some information.

Try journalling the emotional responses you felt from doing a certain task and set goals for what you would like to do in the next day, week, month, or year. Looking forward to something in the future is necessary for all of us to keep going.

Overall, if you don't use it, you'll lose it. This goes for cardio exercise, resistance training, sexual intercourse, and brain and balance exercises equally. Having balance is one of the key fall prevention strategies. You should aim to do this activity on a daily basis if you can, as it doesn't cost money and it can be done anywhere.

As the Nike corporation has said in the past, "Just Do It."

SAMPLE BRAIN TRAINING PROGRAM

WEEK	M	T	W	T	F	S	S
1	MEDITATE 20 MINUTES		JOURNALING 20 MINUTES		SHOP WITH MENTAL MATH 20 MINUTES		
2		CROSSWORD/ SUDOKU/ WORD SEARCH 20 MINUTES		DANCING 1 HOUR		CRAFTS 1 HOUR	
3	CARDS 1 HOUR		LEARN A NEW ACTIVITY		SOCIALIZE WITH FRIEND 1 HOUR		
4		CRAFT 1 HOUR		MEDITATE 20 MINUTES		GAMES 1 HOUR	

CHAPTER SUMMARY

Balance and brain training can be initiated at any time and for any fitness level. Once you make an effort to incorporate some of these gentle activities into your life, you'll feel accomplished and will be more confident and ready to add in other activities noted in this book such as, range of motion, light resistance, and then cardio regimens as your body tolerates.

Remember, *any* activity is better than *no* activity, so do what you can.

CHAPTER 8:
COMBINING ROUTINES AND ACTIVITY PLANS FROM CHAPTERS 4-7

In Chapter 6, we reviewed the basic concepts of weight and resistance training, and there is a plethora of available literature to further your own education by reading, watching YouTube videos, and looking things up on the Internet. If you're not technologically savvy, ask a friend or family member for assistance to find what you're looking for.

While I think that basic balance exercise, range of motion exercises, and low-grade cardio can be initiated all together, I would very slowly incorporate the resistance training so as not to overwhelm yourself and your muscle groups. Sometimes too much change at once is difficult to process. The resistance training can be started on one of the two days you're not doing your cardio, after you have firmly established your routine of cardio, balance, range of motion for at least two weeks. At the earliest, week three or four is when you should be able to move from your range of motion activities to more resistance exercises or weight training. The key here is to start very slowly and not overload your muscle groups. The old adage "no pain no gain" doesn't apply, especially if we're older or deconditioned. A workout should engage your muscles to the point that they let you know that they've been worked a day or two later, but you shouldn't be incapacitated with pain. We don't want to burden your muscles to the point of full muscle exhaustion, as that's not necessary nor is it a safe way to exercise as we get older. If we do have balance issues and/or "dropsy," then perhaps weight machines would be a better option for those who are off-balance and/or clumsy. Again, none of these regimens are suggested to make you feel worse.

After four weeks of reasonable progressive activity, most people will find a benefit in their sleep, psychological status, blood pressure control, blood glucose control, sex life, improved fatigue, and general well-being. It does take at least four weeks to see these benefits, so compliance and persistence will be challenges to overcome, once motivation has been successfully conquered.

There is no one complete set of rules for exercise with resistance as we get older. The basic premise is that if you're going to work one muscle group, you need to do equal work on the opposite muscle group to maintain balance. Again, the suggestions in this book are the basic things that I do on a regular basis that have provided me with success. Every individual client needs to individualize their exercises. There is a need to have functional strength and mobility as we get older. For example, in my very unfit years preceding this last year or two, I loved to have a bath. I noticed that due to deconditioning and excessive weight, I was having difficulty lifting my large butt out of the bathtub with my arm strength at the time. While this was one of the several factors that caused me to change my activity levels, I certainly felt a lot older than my stated age. I remember having to get on all four limbs in the bathtub and keep the water in the tub for buoyancy to get myself out. What a sight! I am so very happy to report that I now do triceps dips while in the tub (but that is not an exercise I would regularly recommend).

When I moved to my condo in Victoria, I noted that there were thirty-four stairs to my unit. It's only been in the last six months that I can sprint up the stairs without any cardiorespiratory limitations. This has taken a lot of work, and eighty pounds less is part of the reason why it's easier. But with improved fitness, endurance, balance, and flexibility, I can do this and many other tasks without any limitations now. Today I was in my garden, cleaning out last fall's debris and weeds. I noticed I was able to get up and down with much more ease that last year. Yes, my knees still creak—I do have some osteoarthritis—but they no longer ache at night with my improved fitness level. I am positive that the leg squats and lunges I've been doing this last year have resulted in a markedly improved ability to get up off the ground. This is an important improvement in safety when I'm gardening alone. We're all at risk of falls (tripping over the garden hose, for example), but being able to mobilize by yourself (unless there's a serious injury, like a broken pelvis or hip) reduces the risk of something else happening *after* you've fallen. Post-fall issues can be caused by a long lie before assistance, hypothermia in cool weather, hyperthermia in hot weather, a raccoon, bear, or cougar coming into yard to see what's up, etc.

When I give a client suggestion on how to incorporate low-level resistance training into their regimen, I highly recommend that they take the time and money to either hire a workout coach or a trainer. The purpose is to get short-term lessons in proper weightlifting techniques or use of machines. An alternative to that would be to seek out a physiotherapist or a kinesiologist privately to help you with the range of motion and other activities. Many clients will tell me, "Karen, I can't afford this." Money has been tight for most people, especially those on fixed incomes, due to the rate of inflation as we come out of the pandemic. However, most of the older adults I know have never prioritized themselves or their health. If we were to ask their families, who love and cherish them, they'd gladly pay for the instructions to help Mom or Dad to be less frail, do the right activities safely, prevent pain and injury, and increase overall well-being. This is the best Christmas gift, birthdate gift, or anniversary gift one can give to older friends and families, especially if the older adult has mentioned this desire and they're motivated to do these activities.

Hopefully, you will get a positive response from your family member that needs more activity. If you feel that your mom or dad needs to improve upon their physical or cognitive fitness or functional status, don't be discouraged if you do not get buy-in right away. The culture of the older age group (early boomers) is that they didn't all necessarily believe in sustaining formal exercise programs as part of their adult and later lives. There are, of course, exceptions to this rule. By and large, especially in rural communities, the life's work in the yard, garden or on the farm was considered, and sometimes still is, to be enough exercise for an individual. I would tend to disagree and have seen this on a regular basis in the stress testing diagnostic labs in my career.

If exercising is a foreign concept to the older adult, gentle nudging, exploration of acceptable activities and SMART goal encouragement will be required in order to increase their activity levels. The local pharmacist, clinic nurse, primary care provider or local trainer may actually be the individuals that have more credibility in convincing the senior to "do just a little bit more." If these older adults are determined not to exercise, then doing some of the bed, chair, brain and balance exercises may be place where families can build on those new activities and then to try something a little more challenging on the physical spectrum. Family members should continue to emphasize the benefits of all these programs and how important it is to prevent frailty and to stay in one's home safely, for as long as possible, if that is the desire of the senior.

There will be times when these exercises for balance, resistance training, or cardio are just too much for an individual. Perhaps that person has been hospitalized recently, or has recently undergone chemotherapy or radiation therapy. Perhaps this individual has severe osteoporosis or osteoarthritis and is extremely frightened that any sort of activity may result in a fall or increase their pain. If this is the case, then the progression to exercise programs may start simply with bed and chair exercise.

The following is a list of gentle bed exercises that can be done in bed, lying flat and without the covers on.[48] Some of these exercises start with appropriately being able to get in and out of bed. If anyone has had abdominal surgery, this is one of the first taught interventions, by the nurses, in order to keep your incision from causing excessive pain in the first few days postoperatively. This includes lowering yourself using your arms and not twisting your back and then bringing up your legs from the side of the bed and gently repositioning yourself.

Other bed exercises can include:

Hips thrusts: Start by lying flat on your back on a mattress without a pillow under your head. Bend your knees and place your feet flat on the mattress as close to your buttocks as you can. While tightening your abdominal muscles and gluteal muscles, slowly press her hips up

---

48 "4 Easy Exercises for Seniors Who Are Bedridden," Home Care Assistance, accessed August 24, 2022, https://www.homecareassistanceparkcities.com/exercises-for-aging-adults-who-are-bedbound/.

toward the ceiling and hold at the top for ten seconds. Then slowly lower down. Repeat eight to twelve times.

Shoulder exercises: Sit cross-legged on the bed and let arms hang loose to the sides. Raise arms straight out beside you until they're at shoulder height and squeeze shoulders at the top. Slowly lower arms back down. Repeat eight to twelve times. Do the same thing with the arms out in front of you, palms facing down. Repeat eight to twelve times.

Hand exercises: Hold a pillow in both hands. Squeeze the pillow tightly with your hands for ten seconds. Repeat eight to twelve times.

Leg lifts: Lie flat on your back without a pillow under your head and with your legs extended out in front of you. Lift feet off the bed toward the midline of your body so that the feet are straight above your hips. Keep your arms close to your side. Then slowly lower your legs. Repeat eight to twelve times. If this is too much, then you can bend the legs at the knees and then straighten your knees. Repeat eight to twelve times.

Foot flexion exercises: Sit up in bed with pillows propped behind you, extend the legs in front of you. Slowly and with control, point toes as far away from your head as you can and then flex back toward your face. Repeat eight to twelve times.

These bed exercises for a week or two, is a gentle way to start an exercise regimen.[49] There are so many to try. We need strong arms for our activities of daily living, strong legs for ambulation and getting up from a chair or toilet, a strong core (abdominal muscles) for balance and chronic back pain, and strong hands to open that darn jar of olives![50]

How does an older adult incorporate ALL of the exercises outline in Chapters 4, 5, 6 and 7?

---

49 Dalia Richmond, "7 Essential Bed Exercises for Elderly," The Geriatric Dietician, accessed August 24, 2022, https://thegeriatricdietitian.com/bed-exercises-for-elderly/.

50 https://www.pensionsweek.com/blog/bed-exercises-for-elderly

It can be overwhelming to take in all these options and decide what to do and when. For simplicity's sake, the next few tables will amalgamate the activities for three fictional individuals.

Class A Activities – for Anne

Anne cannot walk a block, cannot climb one flight of stairs, has severe COPD and is very short of breath with any activity.

	BRAIN	BALANCE	ROM	ROM	ROM	CARDIO		PROGRESS
WEEK	BRAIN	BALANCE*	BED	CHAIR	RESISTANCE	CARDIO	COMMENTS	
& 2	2-3 ACTIVITIES PER WEEK	COUNTER BALANCING ONE LEG AT A TIME	A 1,2	NONE	NONE	NONE	*BALANCE EXERCISES ONLY IF SUPERVISED	
& 4	2-3 ACTIVITIES PER WEEK	ABOVE PLUS LEG LIFTS	A 3,4	NONE	NONE	NONE		
–8	2-3 ACTIVITIES PER WEEK	ABOVE PLUS CLOSING EYES	A 5-8	NONE	NONE	NONE		
–12	2-3 ACTIVITIES PER WEEK	ABOVE PLUS MOVING ARMS	A 9-12+	NONE	NONE	NONE		
3+	2-3 ACTIVITIES PER WEEK	ABOVE PLUS RECITING ALPHABET	A 9-12+	LIGHT 1 LB DUMBBELLS FOR BICEPS AND TRICEPS SQUATS IN AND OUT OF CHAIR	NONE	NONE	8-12 REPETITIONS ONE SET FOR WEEK 13 AND INCREASE BY 2 SETS WEEKS 14, 15	CAN GO ONTO CLASS B ACTIVITIES AFTER WEEK 13 IF STABLE

BRAIN TRAINING EXERCISES A, B, OR C GROUPS: CHOOSE ANY OF THE ACTIVITIES IN THE CHART BELOW

Sample Brain Training Program:

WEEK	M	T	W	T	F	S/S	S
1	MEDITATE 20 MINUTES		JOURNALING 20 MINUTES		SHOP WITH MENTAL MATH 20 MINUTES		
2		CROSSWORD/ SUDOKU/ WORD SEARCH 20 MINUTES		DANCING 1 HOUR		CRAFTS 1 HOUR	
3	CARDS 1 HOUR		LEARN A NEW ACTIVITY		SOCIALIZE WITH FRIEND 1 HOUR		
4		CRAFT 1 HOUR		MEDITATE 20 MINUTES		GAMES 1 HOUR	

BED EXERCISES WEEKS 1 AND 2:

Neck and Back (Sitting in Bed)	Arms and Shoulders (Sitting in Bed)	Legs (Lying in Bed)	Core/Abdomen
gentle flexion and extension of neck and back 8–12 rx1	forward, lateral flexion; lift arms above head; scratch mid back; do up bra 8–12 each activity rx1	straight leg raise, bend knee to chest, side lying clam shell; side lying adductor lifts 8–12 each activity on each leg rx1	none

BED EXERCISE WEEKS 3 AND 4:

as above 8–12 rx2	as above 8–12 rx2	as above 8–12 rx2	planks in bed; leg raises (supine position, lift legs straight up, bend at knee and slowly extend legs without touching mattress) 8–12 r x1

BED EXERCISES WEEKS 5–8:

as above 8–12 rx3	as above 8–12 rx3	as above 8–12 rx3	as above 8–12 rx2

BED EXERCISES WEEKS 9–12+:

as above 8–12 rx3	as above 8–12 rx3	as above 8–12 rx3	as above 8–12 rx3

Class B Activities – for Bob

Bob can walk for 5–10 minutes, can climb one flight of stairs, sometimes has shortness of breath or palpitations when exerting himself mildly. He has angina (chest pain) when really exerting himself.

	BRAIN	BALANCE	ROM	ROM	ROM	CARDIO
WEEK	BRAIN	BALANCE	BED	CHAIR	RESISTANCE	CARDIO
& 2	2-3 ACTIVITIES PER WEEK	COUNTER BALANCING ONE LEG AT A TIME	IF SO DESIRED	IF SO DESIRED	ROM ONLY	BASIC CARDIO EXERCISE PRESCRIPTION 2 FOR CLASS B ACTIVITIES FOLLOW LIST BELOW
& 4	2-3 ACTIVITIES PER WEEK	ABOVE PLUS LEG LIFTS	IF SO DESIRED	IF SO DESIRED	ADD IN 1 LB WEIGHTS OR RESISTANCE TUBING	
–8	2-3 ACTIVITIES PER WEEK	ABOVE PLUS CLOSING EYES	IF SO DESIRED	IF SO DESIRED	ADD IN 2 LB WEIGHTS AND RESISTANCE TUBING	
–12	2-3 ACTIVITIES PER WEEK	ABOVE PLUS MOVING ARMS	IF SO DESIRED	IF SO DESIRED	ADD IN 3 LB WEIGHTS AND RESISTANCE TUBING	
3+	2-3 ACTIVITIES PER WEEK	ABOVE PLUS RECITING ALPHABET YOGA/TAI CHI	IF SO DESIRED	IF SO DESIRED	ADD IN 5 LB WEIGHTS AND RESISTANCE TUBING	

BASIC CARDIO EXERCISE PRESCRIPTION #2 FOR CLASS B ACTIVITIES

* If unhealthy/deconditioned/out of shape/heart disease/CHF/ uncontrolled hypertension etc.

	Warm up	Target heart rate (70%) Minutes per session in THR zone	EXERTIONAL SCALE 1-10	Progression (pace = walking like you're late for an appointment)	Cool down	Frequency	Incline If using treadmill
Week 1	5 mins	3–5	2–3	Increase THR by ½–1 min each session	5 mins	3Xweek	0
Week 2	5 mins	5–11	2–3	Increase THR ½–1 min per session	5–6 mins	5Xweek	0
Week 3	5 min	11–18	3–4	Increase THR ½–1 min per session	6–7 mins	5Xweek	0
Week 4	5 mins	18–23	3–4	Increase THR ½–1 min per session	10 mins	5Xweek	0
Week 5–8	5 mins	23–28	4–6	Increase THR ½–1 min per session	10 mins	5Xweek	0
Week 9–12	5 mins	28–32	4–6	Increase THR ½–1 min per session	10 mins	5Xweek	1–4% grade
Week 12+	5 mins	>30	5–7	At 150 mins per week	10 mins	5Xweek	5% + as desired/ tolerated

Class C Activities – for Carole

Carole can walk 40–60 minutes, can climb several flights of stairs, and has no medical issues when exerting herself.

	BRAIN	BALANCE	ROM	ROM	ROM	CARDIO
WEEK	BRAIN	BALANCE	BED	CHAIR	RESISTANCE	CARDIO
1 & 2	2–3 ACTIVITIES PER WEEK	COUNTER BALANCING ONE LEG AT A TIME	IF SO DESIRED	IF SO DESIRED	ROM AS WARM UP THEN 2–5 LB WEIGHTS AND RESISTANCE TUBING	SEE BELOW BASIC CARDIO PRESCRIPTION 1 FOR CLASS C ACTIVITIES FOLLOW LIST BELOW
3 & 4	2–3 ACTIVITIES PER WEEK	ABOVE PLUS LEG LIFTS	IF SO DESIRED	IF SO DESIRED	AS ABOVE	
5–8	2–3 ACTIVITIES PER WEEK	ABOVE PLUS CLOSING EYES YOGA/TAI CHI	IF SO DESIRED	IF SO DESIRED	AS ABOVE 5–8 LBS WEIGHTS AND RESISTANCE TUBING	
9–12	2–3 ACTIVITIES PER WEEK	ABOVE PLUS MOVING ARMS YOGA/TAI CHI	IF SO DESIRED	IF SO DESIRED	AS ABOVE 8–10 LB WEIGHTS AND RESISTANCE TUBING	
13+	2–3 ACTIVITIES PER WEEK	ABOVE PLUS RECITING ALPHABET YOGA/TAI CHI	IF SO DESIRED	IF SO DESIRED	AS ABOVE 10+ LB WEIGHTS IF DESIRED AND RESISTANCE TUBING	

BASIC CARDIO EXERCISE PRESCRIPTION #1 FOR CLASS C ACTIVITIES

* If **healthy**/no heart disease/CHF/uncontrolled hypertension/etc.

	Warm up	Target heart rate (85%) Minutes per session in THR zone	EXERTION SCALE	Progression (pace = walking like you're late for an appointment)	Cool down	Frequency	Incline If using treadmill
Week 1	5 mins	3–5	4–6	Increase THR by 1–2 minutes each session	5 mins	3Xweek	0
Week 2	5 mins	11–21	4–6	Increase THR 1– 2 mins per session	5–6 mins	5Xweek	0
Week 3	5 min	21–25	4–7	Increase THR 1–2 minutes per session	6–7 mins	5Xweek	0
Week 4	5 mins	25–35	5–7	At THR time; increase duration if weight loss required	10 mins	5Xweek	0
Week 5–8	5 mins	30–35	6–8	At THR time; increase duration if weight loss required	10 mins	5Xweek	3–5% grade
Week 9–12	5 mins	30–35	6–8	At THR time; increase duration if weight loss required	10 mins	5Xweek	5–10% grade
Week 12+	5 mins	30–35	6–9	At THR time; increase duration if weight loss required	10 mins	5Xweek	10% + as desired

CHAPTER SUMMARY

How do you incorporate all this new exercise and brain training information into your life?

At any point in reading this book, you can choose to follow any of the ideas for cardio, resistance training, brain, bed, chair, and balance exercise individually or all together. You should only tackle what you are willing to try first. This book can be used as a reference to add in activities if you are not wanting the input of a trainer, coach, physiotherapist, kinesiologist or other activity professional.

Really, there is no right or wrong way to incorporate any of these ideas. If you've been an absolute couch potato, you could start with Activity Class A. If you are uncertain that you will tolerate a full-blown regimen, then start with Activity Class B. Finally, if you already walk regularly or do other work outs regularly and you are not concerned about any pre-existing health conditions, then you can start a program using Activity Class C. If you find any workload too much, back off, slow down and seek out professional or medical assistance if needed. Again, any movement and activity are better than no movement or activity at all. Good luck to all!

CHAPTER 9:
PREPARATION FOR ACTION IN THE FIFTIES—MAYA AND HER MOTHER MARIA

40 is the old age of youth; 50 is the youth of old age. —Victor Hugo[51]

Clinical scenario:

Maya is a fifty-two-year-old menopausal woman who is five-feet-two-inches tall and weighs 125 pounds. She has no active medical issues and considers herself healthy. Because she has been slender all her life, she doesn't follow any formal exercise program. She was a smoker from the age of thirty to forty-two years. Her father passed away at the age of seventy with COPD from smoking, and her mother (Maria) is alive at eighty years of age with diabetes, hypertension, obesity (BMI 38, ideal body weight 72 kg), atrial fibrillation, and chronic kidney disease. Maya has chosen to move in with Maria, as she has been the only child and never married. Maya will move into Maria's home where Maria has lived for the past fifty years.

GENERAL HEALTH CONSIDERATIONS FOR MAYA

Given her smoking history, age and slender body, Maya is at an increased risk of osteoporosis and fragility fractures. Maya could be screened for osteoporosis with a DEXA scan. Because she quit smoking only ten years ago, consideration should be given for screening of a low-dose CT scan of the thorax to rule out lung cancer, as well a routine mammography, pap smears, and screens for colon cancer as local jurisdictions/guidelines suggest. As Maya doesn't have a primary care provider, she needs to put herself on a waiting list or health registry to obtain primary health care in the future. She would benefit from periodically checking her own BP with Maria's machine to be certain she isn't developing asymptomatic hypertension. Her mother is diabetic. I would encourage Maya to periodically check

---

51 Hugo, Victor famous French Novelist and poet.

her blood sugars with her mom's glucometer as she does not have access to primary care. Maya will need to look after herself. As menopause can be challenging for some women, joining a support group may be beneficial. As mood disorders can occur at this time of life, Maya should do an online depression assessment and if positive for depression, could access assistance using her work insurance benefits or employee assistance program. If her depression is severe, accessing care is necessary. Making the most of her appointment with a new provider would include having her medical and surgical history documented for the clinician, having an accurate list of medications and allergies, and having her objective depression assessment available for the clinician to document the pre-treatment score. Being proactive in securing clinician follow-up and community mental health input is key if depression is present.

ACTIVITIES PLAN FOR MAYA

When I look at this clinical scenario, I see a very typical fifty-two-year-old who hasn't been required to exercise to maintain her weight throughout her adult life. In this client population, it's difficult to get somebody to change their opinion and desire to exercise if they've never had a weight issue. I find clients either love or hate exercise. Those that do love exercise can be easily convinced to increase their cardiovascular regimen to the 150 minutes per week in their target heart rate range (eighty-five percent of age-predicted maximum). Maya would benefit from Class C activities as identified in the last chapter. Enthusiastic clients can also be encouraged to initiate additional strength training as well as balance exercises. The benefits of exercise will also help promote less incidence of fragility fractures, as exercise does have a beneficial effect on increasing bone mass. While Maya's metabolic rate hasn't started to slow as yet, our bodies are programmed to gain about five pounds of weight each year, unless we reduce our intake or increase our exercise. All stomachs and butts will increase in size as we age, as will noses and ears, just like we will get wrinkles and our hair will turn white or grey. That may be enough motivation for Maya!

If Maya *hates* exercising, then as a coach, I would have to find a benefit that Maya can identify with. It could be maintaining ideal body weight as one ages, as her metabolism does slow down, or prevention of those osteoporotic fractures given her smoking history and small body frame. She may need to look at her family history of diabetes and may be worried about becoming diabetic, like her mom, with a lot of chronic comorbidities. The risk for diabetes will increase with advancing age and increasing weight.[52] Whatever the discussion, Maya has to buy in to something that *she decides* is the reason to change. And it will positively benefit her in the long run.

If I had an estimate of her cardiac capacity (like a formal exercise treadmill test), we could talk about how she did at that time. If we don't have that information, I'd start by suggesting that she go out most days of the week and start a walking regimen. The first week should be a walk at a brisk pace after a five-minute warmup for the amount of time she can do a brisk walk with a five-to-ten-minute cool down. Each week, she should increase her brisk walking time so that she's briskly walking thirty minutes daily at the end of the month. I find that clients with an Apple watch, Fitbit monitor, or other heart rate device can easily track their heart rate, and the fifty-two-year-old target heart rate is 134–152 bpm. While it's difficult to get the heart rate up that high with just walking, some options include adding in ankle and wrist weights, increasing the arm movement with walking, walking up hills throughout part of the walk, or periodically doing a short spurt of running or ten to fifteen jumping jacks to get the heart rate elevated into the target zone. One can also chose activities such as treadmill walking with incline, swimming, biking, aerobics, skiing, dancing, skipping rope, step aerobics, or anything that's easy on the joints and can be done most days of the week. The Class C activity plan in Chapter 8 is a good reference for Maya.

---

52 R. Paul Robertson and Miriam S. Udler, "Pathogenesis of Type 2 Diabetes Mellitus," UpToDate, accessed August 24, 2022, https://www.uptodate.com/contents/ pathogenesis-of-type-2-diabetes-mellitus?search=diabetes%20 mellitus&source=search_result&selectedTitle=12~150&usage_type=default&display_ rank=9#:~:text=Subclassification%20based%20on,other%20populations%20 %5B43%5D.

It is important to note that you don't have to continue with only one exercise modality. These aerobic exercises can be mixed and matched and managed according to what is available for the client during the week. A pass to the local gym is only of value if you're truly going to use it. Other benefits of a gym pass are access to proper training and instruction on weight machines and other non-cardio activities, as well as getting in social interactions on a regular basis. It's important for all people to realize that going to the gym or exercising isn't about how we look. If appearances change or weight reduces, then that's a beneficial side effect. The goal of cardio exercise is to have long-standing cardiovascular fitness as we get older. Exercise is not for vanity; it's for longevity and safety.

Once Maya is happy with her cardiac workload, in a few weeks I would prescribe low resistance weight training exercises to improve her arm strength, shoulder strength, core strength, and leg strength. While this may be done at the local gym, purchasing a small set of dumbbells for your arm and shoulder workouts is relatively inexpensive, and then these exercises can be done at home. Leg and core exercises are available from the Internet, but basically include exercises such as squats, lunges, leg lifts, and core exercises, such as planks. Paying for a trainer to give you a basic workout for these key areas in a proper format will let you sustain and then progress in your workouts with a lower risk of injury. Of course, the Internet has many self-guided tutorials on how to work out any part of one's body, and many clients have family members who are also active at the gym.

As we age, our ability to balance decreases. Unlike children who play hopscotch and balance on fences, beams, or any other part of the house or yard their parents don't want them to practise balancing on, as we age, we need to practise balancing. I recommend some simple exercises at the kitchen sink. Stand with your feet shoulder-width apart and put your hands out fully extended at the side. Then stand there with eyes open, and then closed for thirty seconds. Knowing that you can grab onto the sink if you get unsteady, you can then repeat this exercise with your feet close together, and eventually with your eyes closed you can bring in your index fingertip and take turns touching the nose with your eyes closed.

Then you can practise standing on one foot alone, with arms by the side and then arms outstretched at the side, then with eyes closed. Repeat on the other side. You'll be surprised at how quickly your balance will improve after you start doing these exercises (that take less than five minutes at the kitchen sink while you're waiting for your coffee to brew in the morning). If you're not able to progress with these balance exercises, then further investigations may be required by your primary care provider. The organ systems involved with balance include feet, joints, peripheral nervous system, spinal cord, brain, inner ear, and eyes.

At any point in her pursuit of fitness, she can add in these balance exercises. Again, Maya would benefit from an exercise prescription for Class C activities as written in the last chapter.

BRAIN ACTIVITIES PLAN FOR MAYA

Because Maya is still actively employed and doesn't feel that she has to actually "look after her mother" right now, she plans to continue working at her current job. She thinks she'll be ready to retire in seven years, but she doesn't have many interests outside of work. She belongs to a bowling league and continues to go bowling twice weekly. She's also interested in learning some new crafts, like knitting, which she can do basically in most environments. She sounds open to trying new activities as her free time permits. The brain activity suggestions in Chapter 7 will help her formulate a brain activity program.

SOCIAL CONCERNS FOR MAYA

The transition from work to retirement will require Maya to increase her social connections. Establishing a network of friends now will allow her some socialization and companionship. If Maria becomes more dependent on Maya for care, Maya will need to maintain these relationships and socialization plans as part of her own self care regimen. Maya is Maria's only family member. She has now moved into Maria's house and is hopeful that her mom doesn't need much for assistance for the next seven years until she retires. Maya will need to review her mother's mental and physical health regularly and will need to know what kind of behaviours or conditions, when present, will trigger the need for her to retire and become a caregiver. Outpatient social workers and community mental health workers may provide insight into when this will occur. Outside care givers may also be more objective when elderly clients are beginning to decline functionally and cognitively. Maya believes that she'll be able to make changes in her life to fit in with the potential caregiving needs of her mom in seven years. She is fully aware of all of Maria's health problems as Maria has been very transparent in sharing her health concerns with her daughter. Maya does not have a functional crystal ball to predict what will happen in the future, but she is realistically aware that at Maria's age and with her comorbid conditions, her overall condition can change suddenly.

Because this mother and daughter duo have decided to cohabitate, this does allow for social interactions for both Maya and her mother. Hopefully, these social interactions are functional and positive for both members of the family. They will need to work out a living agreement that includes cohabitation rules and guidelines. One of the most important things about the cohabitation agreement is the timing of the completion of this agreement. This ideally should be done well ahead of moving in together. Psychological safety is just as important in your home as in your office or work setting. When having family conversations, there has to be mutual respect and equal opportunities to voice any concerns. Each participant in the home has to have social sensitivity and empathy, as these women, even though they're close family members, grew up in different eras and process information differently. They need to show each other unconditional respect. The ground rules should also set out that blaming one another for certain things that happen in the home is counterproductive and should be replaced with curiosity, so as not to assign blame to the other one in sensitive conversations. Finally, we are all human and we don't choose our family. We need to give each other the grace and space to make mistakes. Maya and Maria will need to refrain from punishing one another or "keeping score" if issues arise.

As Maria ages, if the relationship is perceived as volatile, Maya's interaction with her mother might be construed by an outsider as emotional, physical, or financial elder abuse. A lawyer may need to get involved with assigning responsibilities of care, especially if there are other siblings available that could be involved with Maria's care. In this scenario, Maya is the only child so this is not necessary. However, formal documentation of financial and medical power of attorney will require a lawyers visit when Maria's will be next reviewed. The cohabitation agreement should clearly set out what Maria and Maya are responsible for paying, and how this financial dynamic will change when Maria needs more care. The cohabitation agreement should be done before they move in together for clarity and to troubleshoot any foreseeable conflicts. Maya should not promise Maria that she will *never* be placed in a long-term care home. This puts unnecessary guilt and pressure on the family members when they determine that behaviours or conditions of the parent cannot be safely tolerated at home by the caregiver(s). The conditions of the home and the cohabitation agreement should provide each member of the household, the equal opportunity for use of shared spaces along with the ability to do "noisy" tasks. Each member in the cohabitation agreement must ensure that open dialogue will be encouraged when discussing any potential conflicts. Maya should make sure that Maria is doing an equal amount of participation in food preparation, serving, and cleanup. Maria should have the opportunity to make decisions on the meal plans equally with Maya. Active entertainment for Maya and Maria, including specified outings or in-home activities and mutual agreement on dinner guest lists and frequencies are critical to successful cohabitation. Both Maya and Maria need a sense of purpose for these living arrangements to be successful.

DIETARY CONSIDERATIONS FOR MAYA

Maya would like to stay at her current body weight, so if she starts an exercise regimen, she may have to increase her overall caloric intake. While her baseline caloric intake may be about 1700 kcal per twenty-four hours to maintain her weight, her calories burned with activities like cardiac exercise regimens, weight training, and balance exercises should be added to her 1700 kcal per day so that she doesn't lose weight with the additional activities. There are many applications (see app store), such as my fitnesspal.com, which can calculate the calories needed to maintain, lose, or gain weight. As a general rule of thumb, I use the calculation of 30 kcal per kilogram of ideal body weight one would like to maintain. Maya can access an outpatient dietician service if she needs more robust education regarding her dietary needs. A general recommendation is to intake a "Mediterranean type" diet with enhanced plant-based foods and less animal meats.

FINANCIAL CONSIDERATIONS FOR MAYA

Financially, Maya is a single woman with no dependents and has never married. When she gets older, she will be considered to be a "kinless senior." As she thinks forward to future and specifically her latter few years of life (age 85+), she has to be concerned about who is going to look after her, if she becomes frail, and how she will afford care in the future? Also, Maya needs to consider herself an upcoming caregiver for Maria, and if Maria needs more care than anticipated, Maya might have to quit her job before her expected retirement date.

Are there any financial resources available for Maya to help look after Maria at this current stage of life?

If Maria obtained long-term care insurance before her age cut-off date (ideally obtained between ages fifty-five and sixty-five), and she has met the criteria for needing care, a claim can be made after the waiting period on the contract has been satisfied. The benefit amount, if approved, would be paid tax-free to Maria for the amount of coverage she had. This money can be used to pay for tax deductible care to reduce taxes on her other taxable income.[53] This equates to more available after-tax income. These products *must* be purchased well in advance of the cut-off age, and waiting periods and benefits

---

53 Must CRA qualifications for tax deductibility for tax emptions

amounts are variable. Affordability is the key factor in deciding which plan is right for the individual. As with all health insurance products, establishing the product at the youngest age possible will yield the most affordable rates. As the population ages, the number of claims for this product will increase. Therefore, this will affect and impact both existing and new policies, with possible increasing premiums going forward. These are complicated concepts and this is *not* an online purchase. My recommendation is that clients will need to discuss these options with your certified financial planner.

If Maya has no income source while looking after her mother and waiting for her pension, what are her options?

If Maria were given an ominous prognosis with a very short lifespan and was considered to be a candidate for palliative care, Maya could at that point, explore using her Employment Insurance options to provide compassionate care.

Usually, Maya would not be able to take income from her pension until at least age fifty-five, and a penalty for early pension use would affect her later in her life by reducing her indexed pension for all future years.

One strategy to consider would be for Maria to pay Maya as a caregiver, a **fair wage** that would allow Maya to have money (as a T4 income) to apply to her future Canadian Pension Plan (CPP). This would also allow Maria to have a tax deduction for caregiving from her retirement income streams and/or long-term care insurance. Assuming Maria gets income from her late spouse's pension, she would also have her own OAS and any CPP income as a survivor's benefit as well.

Maya, being single with no dependants, and seeing how much help her mom potentially needs, could also consider long-term care insurance for herself. She is overall healthy and young enough that she may qualify, and it would be more affordable than waiting until she's older. As Maya needs to worry about her future, she should invest as much as she can afford (either while still working or after being paid by her mom) into her Tax Free Savings Account (TFSA) investment plan.

She likely doesn't need to reduce taxes by using the tax deferral of an Registered Retirement Savings Plan (RRSP) and would benefit more from compound growth tax-free, if her income is in the lower tax bracket as a caregiver. A scenario such as this would be:

> $500 per month earning a long-term return rate of five percent would generate a growth to $76,464.31 by age sixty-five for Maya. She could then turn that into tax-free income, with her advisor, of at least $382 per month, plus getting her Old Age Security (OAS) at sixty-five and electing her CPP at that age to avoid reductions. Her pension could then be elected at sixty-five without penalty, or possibly earlier if bridging is available. She would have direct benefit pension options at age sixty and beyond (she could choose at any time), depending on the pension options and if there is bridging. She could even elect early.

What can Maya do to look after Maria if Maya falls ill and passes away before her mother?

Maya should have life insurance to support Maria if she dies, and critical illness insurance should be procured in case Maya falls ill and can't work (income protection). She should review her work group insurance plan for convertibility of both life and critical illness products ***before* she retires or leaves work**. Maya's last will and testament should leave everything to Maria if Maya predeceases her, and she should consider establishing a professional executor (CFP or lawyer) to decrease the burden of estate duties on an elderly Maria.

How can Maya maintain her benefits if she needs to quit her job or retire? There are two possible options. The first is to consider purchasing personal health insurance if she has no medications or pre-existing medical conditions. Second, if she does have health issues requiring treatments or medications, a conversion to a "no evidence" group, which must be completed within a short time frame of leaving work (thirty days), will offer her coverage for pre-existing and new conditions but with lower coverage amounts and slightly higher costs when compared to the "evidence" purchased, personal health insurance in the first option.

ADVOCACY CONSIDERATIONS FOR MAYA

From an advocacy point of view, Maya is still working and will be a caregiver for her mom. In Canada, there are more than 7.8 million people providing care for someone at home. As a vested caregiver in our society, Maya needs to be certain that services, such as adequate home care and home supports are available when the time comes that she needs help with her mom. Maria is still competent and has no evidence of dementia yet. While there are things she can do to improve her physical health, social isolation for Maria would be extremely detrimental going forward. Maria and friends or family members in a similar age group will need to make sure that their social interactions are maintained, and elders can and should advocate for increased services for seniors. Joining like minded individuals in groups like seniors helping seniors, promoting improved access to day programs such as adult or geriatric day hospital, and/or community exercise and entertainment programs can be initiated at any point in time. There is no time like the present to start advocating for future care as we age.

The Office of the Seniors Advocate is an independent office of the BC Provincial Government. It acts in the interest of seniors and their caregivers and has a toll-free number: 1–877–952–3181 and website: www.seniorsadvocatebc.ca. This office monitors the senior services and makes recommendations to the government and service providers to address systemic issues in the areas of healthcare, housing, income support, community support, and transportation. There are a number of provincial and local organizations that help with advocacy issues for seniors, including legal advocacy. Those details can be found on the website www.seniorsfirstbc.ca. CARP is heavily invested in advocating for home care and elder care in general. Joining a local chapter of CARP may provide more insight to Maya as both she and her mother get older.

The next few paragraphs will be the recommendations for the matriarch of this fictional family, Maria.

GENERAL HEALTH CONSIDERATIONS FOR MARIA

It is in Maya's best interest that Maria starts an age-appropriate exercise program, continues with good self-care of her diabetes, hypertension, and atrial fibrillation, gets on an ideal weight management program, and avoids medications or treatments that could worsen chronic kidney disease. Her primary care provider should have given her medications specifically to help her blood pressure and protect her kidneys given her diabetes and hypertension. Her glycemic control needs to be monitored, but given her age, she may be better off to have a higher hemoglobin A1c so that she doesn't experience any episodes of hypoglycemia. Being a diabetic with chronic kidney disease, currently her goal blood pressure would be under 130/80. Her eye exams need to be done every six to twelve months, including a retinal examination to rule out diabetic and hypertensive retinal damage that may affect her vision down the road. Quarterly blood work is the standard of care for diabetics, and it looks at glycemic control, basic chemistry, and renal parameters. Liver function tests should be performed, as at Maria's current weight and with her comorbid conditions, she's at high risk of developing fatty liver disease. Maria may need age-appropriate cancer investigations depending on the development of any new or concerning symptoms. Given Maria's age, certain medications such as anticholinergic medications or sedatives should be avoided, as they could have a detrimental effect on cognition and could double the risk of falls and fractures. At this age, she is currently not in the age category for screening for most of the common cancers but should seek out urgent health care if she develops any constitutional symptoms such as fevers, night sweats, unintentional weight loss, easy bleeding or bruising, new blood loss from the gastrointestinal or genitourinary systems. If primary health care is not available, a visit to an urgent care centre may be required. As a last resort, a visit to the emergency room may be required to facilitate an urgent work up for these potentially ominous symptoms but this is NOT IDEAL for long term care and follow-up.

ACTIVITIES PLAN FOR MARIA

I would definitely recommend that Maria have cardiac exercise testing prior to starting any aggressive exercise regimen, as her pre-test probability for heart disease would be high and her chance of having a heart attack in the next ten years would be in excess of forty percent.[54] With cardiac exercise testing and being sure that there is no need for urgent medical or other interventions, she may start on a exercise regimen, but unlike Maya's exercise plan, Maria should start with either Class A or B activities as suggested in Chapter 8. Maria's blood pressure and heart rate response with the atrial fibrillation and medications may limit the overall amount of workload that Maria can do. In this situation, I would be satisfied with Maria doing thirty minutes of a Karen Perceived Exertion Score of 3–5 in either Class A or Class B activities. The benefit of doing exercise for Maria would include her potential to develop collateral circulation in her coronary arteries if she already has some development of blockages in the large or small vessels of the heart.

A similar light-weight regimen and balance program could be taught to Maria by Maya when Maria was ready for advancement in her activity plan.

BRAIN ACTIVITIES PLAN FOR MARIA

Maria could join Maya and start doing brain activities at any point in time. This could be a nice social outing for the two if a new craft class was started or friends of both women came over to quilt. Maria may have skills such as sewing, knitting, painting, or other artistic skills that should be encouraged on a regular basis. Group outings with similar-aged friends should be encouraged. Meditation, brain puzzles, and other cognitive tasks (mental math when grocery shopping) should be encouraged. Chapter 7 has outlined many potential

---

54 Ralph B. D'Agostino et al, "General Cardiovascular Risk Profile for Use in Primary Care: The Framingham Heart Study," PubMed.gov, January 22, 2008, https://pubmed. ncbi.nlm.nih.gov/18212285/.

skills that can be added to one's weekly schedule for enhancing brain exercise and promoting neuroplasticity.

SOCIAL CONCERNS FOR MARIA

Maria needs to maintain her own social circle outside of Maya's. Each woman in the household needs peer-age companions to socialize with and to provide a safe sounding board for when home life is challenging. Maria should strive for an active social calendar one to three days per week outside of medical appointments and tests. Maria will need to balance her exercise program with household duties and socialization. Maria should listen to her body and rest on days when her body is telling her it's required. If her workouts are too grueling, she should consider starting in a stretch and strength exercise program or local geriatric day hospital program.

DIETARY CONSIDERATIONS FOR MARIA

Maria should be referred to a dietitian for a carbohydrate-controlled diet. I usually recommend under 100g of carbohydrates per day with diabetes (this has worked well for many of my clients) and a daily 2,100-calorie diet that is low in salt and heart-healthy. Canada food guide can also be followed and the overall recommendations for most clients with diabetes is somewhere between 50-70 grams of carbohydrates with meals. Given her atrial fibrillation, she should abstain from alcohol. Given her obesity, her primary care provider also needs to review diabetic medications and optimize those medications that are weight neutral or promote weight loss in addition to being beneficial for the heart and kidneys (such as Jardiance, Semaglutide, metformin, etc.). The Canadian Cardiovascular Harmonized National Guideline Endeavor (C-CHANGE) for the prevention and management of cardiovascular disease in primary care: 2022 update, is a comprehensive resource for primary health care practitioners.[55] This document is

---

55 Jain et al; CMAJ, November 7, 2022; Volume 194, Issue 43 pages E1460-1480. www.cmaj.ca

intended for clinicians but can be used as a resource for many until the next guideline updates are available which occurs every few years.

FINANCIAL CONSIDERATIONS FOR MARIA

Maria may also, if needed, use her paid-for home as a source of cash to provide finances for Maya and herself. Potential options include a reverse mortgage, which allows her to stay and live in the home but reduces the value of her estate, which Maya may eventually need, especially if she was going to take off work and pension building time to look after her mom. Maria may also get a secured line of credit. This benefit also reduces the estate value, but it does usually cost less interest than reverse mortgage. It does require, at the very least, interest payments.

In addition, Maria should add Maya to the title for the home to make the transition upon Maria's death easier for Maya. Also, Maya should have joint bank accounts with Maria so that the funds won't be frozen when Maria dies. Maya can then use the account to continue covering taxes and household bills. In addition, when Maria is no longer able to make decisions, a Power of Attorney (POA) would allow Maya to continue to keep Maria's best interests going forward using Maria's financial resources.

Maria has her spouse's survivor pension, but what happens to that money when she passes away? This money will vanish once Maria passes away, and there will be a one-time CPP death benefit no greater than $2,500, as of today.[56]

What are the legal processes for getting medical and financial power of attorney? This requires seeking out your lawyer while completing or updating your will. Your lawyer will assist in completing legal documents for both Financial and Medical Power of Attorney and decision-making processes.

Under what circumstances does a public trustee become involved? If Maya passes away before Maria, or Maya has no cognitive ability to make decisions for Maria, then social work involvement in a hospital

---

56 Service Canada will determine based on your qualifications.

or community setting will need to liaise with Maria's primary care provider to start the process of getting Public Trustee involvement. This may vary provincially, and your lawyer and social worker can advise the best process for procuring this safety net.

What is a professional executor? These are available professionals (lawyer, notary, other professionals). In British Columbia, this service is governed by the Trustee Act of British Columbia. See the government website under "Wills and Estates." Please refer to your local provincial programs/local jurisdictions in other parts of the world for details. While you can appoint anyone as an executor, a professional executor will deal with *all* estate issues in event that an adult doesn't want to burden their family (or has no family) with this task, especially with complex family dynamics, professional corporations, real estate, or other complicated life circumstances.

ADVOCACY CONSIDERATIONS FOR MARIA

Currently, Maya is Maria's advocate. They have a close personal relationship, and Maria feels very comfortable that when the time comes that she can no longer make medical or financial decisions, Maya will become her POA. She has full trust in Maya. It's never too soon for her to draw up those documents with her lawyer, so that if anything happens to Maria, Maya is able to financially deal with all the processes associated with the death of her mom. Exploring what matters to Maria and helping her advocate for things she is interested in and that will help her in her future, is a reasonable goal to try to achieve. Some seniors don't want to look too far ahead, or even admit to the possibility of institutionalization. Family and caregivers need to respect the senior's decision not to engage in those discussions if it makes them feel uncomfortable. Exploring why there is some discomfort with those discussions may be helpful in order to move discussions along going forward.

If at all possible, having clear directions for care (resuscitative status, medical scope of treatment, or health care directives) needs to be documented by the primary care provider in a clinic setting and reviewed at each hospital admission. BC has the pamphlet *My Voice*[57] available to help clients and their families navigate through these difficult conversations.

REFLECTION AND DISCUSSION:

This scenario is reflective of the middle-aged adult who likely needs to become a caregiver in the future. This has many implications from a general and preventative health perspective, but also there are social, financial, and advocacy concerns identified. This case is a mere example of how forward thinking and planning are required to deal with our uncertain futures while we age. As mentioned, the financial advice given has been reviewed by a certified financial planner, and there are a lot of other circumstances that your own financial planner will need to extensively review. Remember, financial health is just as important and contributes to emotional, psychological and physical health and should be reviewed annually along with your other health interests.

---

57 Government of British Columbia, "My Voice: Expressing My Wishes for Future Health Care Treatment," accessed August 24, 2022, https://www.health.gov.bc.ca/library/publications/year/2013/MyVoice-AdvanceCarePlanningGuide.pdf.

CHAPTER 10:
PREPARATION FOR ACTION IN THE SIXTIES—DEBORAH'S CASE

We are what we repeatedly do. Excellence then, is not an act, but a habit.
—Aristotle

Clinical Scenario:

Deborah is a sixty-four-year-old registered nurse who has been working for the last forty years and plans to retire in the next two months. She has hypertension, is five-feet-four-inches tall, and weighs 215 pounds. Deborah hasn't been physically fit for the last ten years. She's a non-smoker but does enjoy a glass of wine five nights a week. She is single and doesn't anticipate finding a partner anytime soon.

GENERAL HEALTH PRINCIPLES FOR DEBORAH

As the ancient philosopher Aristotle has said, "we are what we repeatedly do. Excellence then, is not an act, but a habit." In Deborah's case, it appears that she has been a life long care giver, working in health care for forty years. It would appear that she may not be the poster child for ideal health and wellness. As she approaches retirement, she has the option of turning her care giving focus from strangers to herself. This is such an opportunity at this time in one's life!

In addition to age-appropriate cancer screening (mammograms, pap smears etc.), Deborah needs to work on trying to become a healthier version of herself, including achieving ideal blood pressure control and attempting to close the gap between current health status and optimal health status. All of the interventions in this book may contribute to a healthier version of Deborah, and this alone could help improve her blood pressure control. She should have all her dental work, eye exams, hearing exams, and any other insurance-covered auxiliary health exams done prior to retiring. A mammogram, pap smear, and screen for colon cancer should ideally all be completed before her union benefits package expires. Many folks retire only to find out that their health is poor and their insurance coverage is gone.

ACTIVITIES PLAN FOR DEBORAH

Deborah would be wise to start with activities Class A or B as outlined in Chapter 8. The first order of business in someone who hasn't been physically active for a very long time would be to start with one week of daily stretching and range of motion exercises. These should be done most days of the week and would include moving the arms forward, sideways, over the head with palms touching each other, scratching the middle of the back, and rotating the arms as if trying to do up a bra. Leg exercises should start with straight leg raises either in bed or in a chair, followed by bent-knee raises. While holding on to a counter, she should extend her leg out and try to bring the heel to touch her buttock. Each of these exercises should be done in repetitions of eight to twelve on both sides: on the first day done once, on the second and third days two sets of eight to twelve repetitions, and after day three, three sets of eight to twelve repetitions for each exercise on each limb. During the second week, gentle walking for at least five to ten minutes at a moderate speed with increasing the length of the walk by one to two minutes every day.

After one month, Deborah should continue with her stretching and walking exercises, but the walking speed is now increased to her fastest tolerable gait. This should happen after a five-minute slow walk warmup. Her thirty minutes of a faster speed is followed by a five-to-ten-minute cool down. This walking should occur five days a week, with each week trying to increase the walking speed of the thirty-minute "power walk."

At the end of the second month, Deborah can add wrist and/ or ankle weights to her walking regimen or add walking sticks or increase her arm motion to try and increase her overall target heart rate to seventy-five to eighty percent of her age-predicted maximum (220 − age). After completing the second month of walking, Deborah may proceed to a more accelerated exercise program with the goal to get her target heart rate to eighty-five percent of her age-predicted maximum for a total of 150 minutes per week (see Chapter 4 - Basic Cardio Exercise Regimen #1).

The basic balance exercises should be undertaken one to three times daily in order to improve overall balance.

For basic weight training exercises for arms (biceps, triceps, shoulders, and chest) and legs (calf raises, hip flexion and extensions, squats, lunges, and planks) see Chapter 6 for details.

BRAIN EXERCISES FOR DEBORAH

Deborah is planning on going back to work after a few months of "retirement" where she hopes to regroup, take better care of herself, and have a more controlled life balance. For her, volunteering in the short-term may help to broaden her scope of potential other jobs, in addition to nursing. Blood pressure treatment with lifestyle modifications and medications, combined with self care are crucial in this next window of life, as she transitions from a full-time employee to a more causal employee. Deborah would be encouraged to initiate any of the brain activities in Chapter 7 and start with doing two or three brain activities each week and challenge herself to learn or try a different activity every 4–8 weeks.

SOCIAL CONCERNS FOR DEBORAH

Deborah has a lot of nursing friends, but she's the only one who's ready to retire. She's not interested in dating and has looked on dating websites, but doesn't feel comfortable in putting herself out there. She needs to be certain that she doesn't get bored at home and increase her drinking. Volunteering and doing crafts may help her during this period. She needs to explore "what makes her happy" and "what makes her feel fulfilled." A purpose for this next phase of life is important to think through. A transition coach may be able to help her with these life changes. As Deborah will be on a fixed income, she must be careful if she does take a new partner into her life. She should consider cohabitation agreements if she finds a partner in the future and they decide to move in together. As her assets are fixed and her work life is essentially finished, consideration of a pre-nuptial agreement would also be suggested if marriage is an option in the future. As with many clients in their later years, sexual activity without the proper protection may place seniors at risk of HIV, syphilis, gonorrhea, chlamydia, herpes, genital warts, and trichomoniasis. Her status as a nurse likely means she has been vaccinated against Hepatitis B, but unprotected intercourse needs to be avoided at all costs until the sexual health of her potential partner has been verified. That being said, the importance of sexual activity in later life in promoting enhanced cardiovascular health, improved self esteem, and elevated quality of level perception need not be deflated with the fear of possibly receiving a sexually transmitted infection. Rather, education and engagement in safe sexual behaviours is the key to promoting a healthy sex life as one ages. In addition, there are many educational sources for solo sex for the senior as well. Overall, orgasms are good for people, and reducing the stigma associated with seniors and healthy sex choices will add quality of life for all those who engage in these activities.

DIETARY CONSIDERATION FOR DEBORAH

If weight loss is desired, I use a formula that gives a client 25 kcal per kilogram of ideal body weight that they want to achieve. If the ideal body weight is 70 kg, then the allotted calorie intake would be 1,750 kcal per twenty-four hours. I would definitely encourage using an app such as "my fitness pal" or "life sum" to help calculate macronutrients (carbohydrates, fats, and proteins) along with overall calories utilized with exercise and consumed during the day. Once you document a month's worth of oral intake, it becomes less of a burden to enter your food because we primarily eat similar things every thirty days.

In order for Deborah to lose weight using exercise alone, she would need to exercise sixty minutes at her target heart rate of eighty-five percent of age-predicted maximum five times a week for a total of at least three hundred minutes of cardio per week or more. That's a lot of cardio, and because weight loss is notoriously unsuccessful, especially as we age, caloric and portion control in addition to a much more manageable 150 minutes of exercise per week seems more reasonable. As alcoholic liquids contain essentially empty calories, I would suggest complete cessation of alcohol in this situation. There is really no current brain or cardiovascular recommendation in the literature that states that drinking alcohol is safe or encouraged.[58] The older studies that looked at heart healthy drinking have been replaced by no recommendations for alcohol for any cardiovascular disease. This is especially true if patients have congestive heart failure or arrhythmias.

From a macronutrient perspective, protein intake is important while building muscle, so in the absence of any significant liver or kidney disease, I would recommend 1 g of protein for each kilogram of ideal body weight per day. While I'm a diabetic with poor carbohydrate tolerance, I tend to recommend limited carbohydrates, which would be those with a low glycemic index and complex carbohydrates with whole grains. Diabetics and those with extra weight on board needs to figure out what kinds of foods affect the weight and/or blood sugars individually. For diabetics, this is easier to achieve if there is at least thirty to sixty days of continuous blood glucose monitoring. For non diabetics, many diets are available to try. More importantly, diets are notoriously unsuccessful and I don't really recommend dieting per se. Long term portion control, carbohydrate counting, and associated lifestyle modifications are going to be better tolerated. The goals are for the individual to choose healthier options over unhealthy options. A robust outpatient dietician service does not always exist in every community. Therefore, guidelines such as using certain portions of protein (like a serving size of protein, equivalent of the size and thickness of the palm of your hand) have been developed. Another simple method is to take one food group each week and cut the portion size by 50%. On week 1, eat 50% less carbs, on weeks 2, eat 50% less carbs and fats and on week 3, if needed, eat 50% less carbs, fats and proteins.

---

58 "One Alcoholic Drink A Day Linked with Reduced Brain Size," PennToday, March 4, 2022, https://penntoday.upenn.edu/news/one-alcoholic-drink-day-linked-reduced-brain-size.

How can Deborah make significant changes all at once? This seems overwhelming, and with retiring, there are too many upcoming changes. While change will be required if Deborah wants to become healthier, it may be daunting. Like everything in life, choices must be prioritized. I would recommend that Deborah take some time for self-reflection to focus on what she wants to accomplish in the next few years. Once those goals are clear, then setting shorter term, more attainable small goals would be next. This is where SMART[59] goal setting is utilized along with traditional pros and cons charts to look at each change required. Adding in changes all at once may not be the best idea.

As Deborah transitions to life as a retiree, it might make sense to start her activity program at a low level before she retires. This way, she won't feel compelled to start everything all at once. She'll need to focus on dealing with the necessary financial decisions so that her finances are prioritized and secured prior to leaving her job. While she's still working, she can slowly incorporate a walking program, and once her work time is complete, she can utilize more free time into the addition of a more robust cardio regimen, adding in balance, brain, and resistance exercises and taking time in her day to express gratitude and enjoy allocated free time.

As with many adults who have attempted to lose weight, it may seem like it will *never* happen. But I can assure you that slow, methodical changes and substituting slightly healthier treats that don't blow your "weight loss budget" will be the start of those lifestyle changes. What Deborah needs to avoid is the "fat shamers" in the world. Even as a physician, I've been treated poorly for being fat. I've had colleagues at meetings look at me and tell me, "Fat people just need to buy fewer groceries." In my physician life, I do know that I have been treated poorly or not taken seriously due to my obesity. When I was a busier clinician, I often would have candid conversations with patients, about diet, weight loss, and diabetes. When I was with patients, I could empathize and acknowledge how difficult the task of

---

59 "Ultimate Guide to SMART Goals," AttendanceBot Blog, May 19, 2020, https://www.attendancebot.com/blog/ultimate-guide-smart-goals/.

successful weight loss really was. I shared those same struggles with clients on a daily basis. There was no fat shaming coming from "the fat specialist," because I understood the challenges and realities of obesity. I would speak of options for the patient to try for a week or two at a time. I was not ignored, at least by my patients in the clinic. I also was not a young, thin physician who had never been less than ideal weight in her entire life. I was a big proponent of choosing fitness first over ideal body weight. These issues with chronically excessive body weight are complex and challenging. Because of this, obesity clinics employ multidimensional professionals who look at the client holistically to deal with the complex processes that contribute to obesity. There are even more complicated pathophysiologic processes in the complications of obesity, which further warrant ongoing specialty team expertise. If you wish more information on obesity medications and interventions, I recommend you liaise with ObesityCanada.ca or contact your primary care provider.

FINANCIAL CONSIDERATIONS FOR DEBORAH

Deborah is about to retire. She's had a full-time job for the last forty years and doesn't have a partner or expect to get one. She has one independent child who lives in another part of the country. She hasn't made a will or obtained a power of attorney.

As Deborah is now working with a certified financial planner. She has received some of the educational resources about retiring from her Human Resources Department at her place of employment. The first educational document she procured and reviewed was "Thinking about Retirement" from the Municipal Pension Plan, which includes her nurses' pension plan. She's also had pre-retirement meetings with the Human Resources Department, and she has also reviewed documents specific to her pension, which includes her generic pension options for funding (cost of living adjustments included/external links to Canada Revenue Agency), taxation of pension guidelines, and extended health care and dental plan extended coverage documents.

Although she hasn't required a lot of medications, she's wondering about possibility of continuing her benefits in retirement. Deborah has reviewed the documents and has made enquiries about purchasing other available personal plans. She is single and finds that the value of her plan, with the reduced cost of staying in her plan, gives exceptional value because of her years of service. If she were married, it would still be good value, but with a spouse (with no service discount) it would not be as exceptional as her single plan. It would still be more affordable than purchasing personal health plans as a couple.

Her certified financial planner will review her pension options for a single person (no surviving benefit), and there will be a discussion about taking a reduced benefit for a guaranteed pension income for a specified period of time. If Deborah had a dependent adult child or was anticipating a new long-term partner, she might consider this, but as a single retiree, she will most likely choose to elect the unreduced maximum pension option, and once elected, it *can't* be changed. As she is not quite sixty-five years of age, she will get bridging, if available, (an amount of money equal to Old Age Secuirty (OAS) and the Canada Pension Plan (CPP) until that time. At that point, she'll contact Service Canada to elect or defer her CPP and OAS. Currently, she is considering casual work in six months' time after taking a well-deserved break from health care.

She may go back to work in six months after she's had some time off to rest. At age sixty-five, if she's still working, she can defer CPP and OAS until age seventy and still gain CPP and OAS benefits by deferring and still working up until the age of seventy. At that time, CPP and OAS must be elected and there will be an extra thirty-six percent OAS and an extra forty-two percent of CPP.[60]

These are options to consider and discuss with one's own certified financial planner and accountant. There will be a tax bracket that Deborah may want to be below so that her extra work isn't all taxed and she still has options to input more RRSPs to offset the tax burden (tax deferred). When she stops working and lowers her income, she'll be able to draw on RRSPs with less tax than if she was still working and in a higher tax bracket.

---

60 Canada Revenue Agency website; CPP and OAS benefits

While she has not yet established a tax free savings account, she will likely be encouraged to open this type of investment account because, as of the publication of this book, she will have $81,500 of contribution room for tax-*free* investment growth and future tax-free income.

Deborah wants to create a legacy fund for her child and grandchildren. She's thinking about taking out and funding a whole life policy on her healthy thirty-two-year-old daughter. It will afford lifetime coverage for her daughter to look after her children and future grandchildren. There will be many years of compounded growth, and Deborah could elect to have this policy paid in full within ten to twenty years. Deborah has opted to purchase a rider on the policy that will ensure that it's paid in full upon her death. While Deborah is alive, she is the owner and her daughter is the contingent owner of the policy, so that if Deborah dies, her daughter is now owner of the paid-up policy.

For her grandchildren, Deborah is electing to set up a family Registered Education Savings Plan (RESP) to provide for all current and future education funding. This investment strategy requires a planner to set up the paperwork to benefit the grandchildren, and requires the parents' signatures to set up. Government grant funding (CESG) applications will be done at the time of opening this investment and will continue to advise as the family grows.

ADVOCACY CONSIDERATIONS FOR DEBORAH

While Deborah is a soon-to-be retired nurse, she has an exquisite knowledge of healthcare over the last four decades and is concerned about the status of long-term care homes in her local community. She is considering volunteering to get a better understanding of the limitations of eldercare in her community and plans on advocating for improved nurse-client ratios as well as affordable housing for seniors who are slightly older than she is.

She may also consider trying to get a job doing private care nursing to explore what options are available for private pay nursing care. She's looking forward to retiring in two months, and after taking some time off to recharge, she's interested in possibly working casually in one of the local personal care homes. She has some concerns about taking on a new job this late in her career. She has read a lot about agism and feels, like many workers in her age group, the some of her younger colleagues have not always been kind to her in her work place. Ageism exists in many organizations in many industries. She is thinking about additional training on conflict resolution to help her deal with the ageism that may be present if and when she adds on a new job to her daily routine. Her goal is to take an online geriatric nursing program during her time off, and with her volunteering at the care home, she'll determine if this location is a good fit for her or not. She only plans on doing one shift per week maximum, as there will be financial implications for this. She was very active in her nursing union and hopes to advocate for less wage discrepancy between hospital and care home nursing pay scales.

REFLECTION AND DISCUSSION:

In this scenario, I reviewed the health and well-being of a soon-to-be retired nurse. There are important health-related recommendations suggested for this stage in her life. I have explored some of the financial considerations that may require a professional review with a financial planner, preferably a certified financial planner. This scenario serves as a topic of discussion for possible scenarios and financial options that one could consider. Financial health, like general health, requires a dedicated professional team to provide the degree of financial care necessary for retirement planning. Please review the diagram in the introduction of this book for details regarding key persons that could be part of your own financial services team.

CHAPTER 11:
PREPARATION FOR ACTION IN THE SEVENTIES

Clinical Scenario:

Virginia and Alicia are good friends. They live several doors down the street from one another and see each other almost daily.

Virginia is seventy-three years of age and is five-feet-eight-inches tall and 160 pounds. She had a heart attack at the age of sixty-eight and required angiogram, angioplasty, two stents in two different arteries, and has congestive heart failure with an ejection fraction of thirty-five percent. She is followed at the local heart function clinic and stopped smoking at the age of sixty-eight when she had her heart attack. She enjoys a glass of wine prior to dinner every night. She has COPD and is on three puffers.

Alicia is Virginia's best friend and is a seventy-nine-year-old female who is five-feet-eight-inches tall and weighs 180 pounds. She has recently been diagnosed with type 2 diabetes and has had high cholesterol for years. She states that she walks daily several blocks and is a non-smoker and a non-drinker. She's had one hip replacement for osteoarthritis and lives alone. She has some family close by but there is limited contact. She has been socially isolated, especially since the COVID-19 pandemic began in 2020.

GENERAL HEALTH RECOMMENDATIONS FOR VIRGINIA

In addition to the usual cancer screening programs in her local health jurisdiction, Virginia should be followed regularly by a primary care provider for her two chronic medical conditions, which are COPD and congestive heart failure with a reduced ejection fraction. While she is followed by her local heart function clinic, this is in a small community and she has no access to a formal cardiac rehabilitation/

exercise program. She has been told that exercise is good for her; however, she needs a more detailed description of what to do. She is compliant with her medications and has them blister-packed for ease of administration. Her heart function specialists adjust her medications every three to six months, and she is aware of her NYHA (New York Heart Association) class symptoms that she tracks on a regular basis. She has never seen a lung specialist for her COPD, and the last time she had a pulmonary function test done was about seven years ago. She quit smoking only five years ago and may be a candidate for a low-dose chest CT scan to screen for lung cancer. She had her hearing tested once in her early sixties and would likely benefit from getting her hearing retested. If she does have a hearing impairment, this can increase the chance of cognitive deterioration.

ACTION PLANS FOR VIRGINIA

Virginia will need a modified exercise regimen for both her COPD and her CHF. She would benefit from an activity program as outlined in Chapter 5, which details some of the modifications of exercise programs, specific for those clients with COPD. She has had ischemic heart disease and has a reduced ejection fraction congestive heart failure (HFrEF). At this stage of her life, Virginia has been frightened to embark on any cardiac rehabilitation routine. She's tried to ask a trainer for advice, but given her heart disease and HFrEF, the trainer at the gym hasn't felt comfortable providing any exercise or weight lifting advice.

As seen in Chapter 8, clients like Virginia can initiate an exercise program using the Class B activities. While Virginia could definitely embark upon an exercise program, such as gentle walking or other low intensity cardiac workouts, her heart rate should be limited to sixty-five to seventy-five percent of her age-predicted maximum (96–110), while her resting heart rate should be between 50–60 bpm. For her congestive heart failure, she will likely be on medications often referred to as goal directed medical therapy (GDMT), which could include diuretics, ace inhibitors/ARBs or ARNIs, beta blockers, MRA medications such as spironolactone, and possibly newer agents that are

SGLT2 inhibitors, now frequently used in type 2 diabetes. With the decreased ejection fraction, these clients are often sodium and fluid restricted during the day, and it's very important for them not to be over hydrated or dehydrated. The exercise regimen should be able to be done comfortably with the goal of working only minimally hard. The reduced pump function of the heart (decreased ejection fraction) can contribute having a lot of symptoms with minimal exertion and can also make this client prone to arrhythmias. Clinicians often advocate for alcohol abstention in this client population. She can certainly attempt Class B activities noted in Chapter 8 but modify the work load if her breathing is too labored. She needs to review her own NYHA class symptoms and mMRC score (Chapter 5). In Virginia's case, excessive breathing troubles could mean a flare up of either her COPD or her CHF. Ideally, Virginia should be followed in a proper cardiac rehab or respiratory rehab program. A less ideal option, would for Virginia to do her work load with a chaperone who has basic life saving training, and only exercise in the presence of that individual, and only in areas where cell phone service and ambulance personnel are available. It is not known if telehealth availability for these types of programs would provide any additional benefit or not. Clinicians do acknowledge that overall, exercise is important in the majority of clients with CHF and COPD alike. It is more reassuring for the client to do this in a supervised program but gentle Class B activities can be attempted.

Virginia can continue with balance exercises and can do a very light weight regimen as long as she doesn't hold her breath or bear down (Valsalva manoeuvre) when she's doing her weights.

If Virginia develops chest pain while doing her activities, she will need to seek medical attention as soon as possible. She would require an evaluation and be cleared, likely by a specialist, to safely return to her exercise program. Once she is cleared (investigations completed and medications adjusted) and can go back to her regimen, she would benefit from returning to exercise, peaking at a lower level, which would be a heart rate approximately 10 bpm lower than the threshold which triggers her chest pain/angina. As mentioned earlier,

Virginia would be best served doing exercises in a supervised cardiac rehabilitation program. Due to her increased risk of arrhythmia, I wouldn't recommend any solo activities or activities such as swimming. Low intensity water exercise classes could be entertained if symptoms don't limit the activity and the facility had an automatic external defibrillator present, should anything should go awry while she is at the facility.

BRAIN EXERCISES FOR VIRGINIA

Virginia and her friend Alicia are active gardeners. They're always looking up plants on the Internet and reviewing the optimal growing conditions for these plants. Both of these women go out for weekly coffee with a group of like-minded friends to discuss current events. When Virginia is alone, she plays cards (solitaire) and does sudoku two to three times a week. She has some computer skills for basic email and texting function. She has been doing a new game, WORDLE, on her computer and comparing her success with her grandsons.

SOCIAL CONCERNS FOR VIRGINIA

When Virginia is online, she has enough knowledge of basic computer skills, but often finds spam emails that she is not sure whether or not these pose a risk to her online privacy. Her family constantly reminds Virginia NOT to click on any links in her text, email, or social media feeds if she is unaware of where the message is coming from. Likewise, her family reminds her that usually financial institutions and the Canada Revenue Agency DO NOT contact people using these forms of communications. All seniors need to have discussions with a computer savvy contact person to be certain that they do not become victims of financial abuse.

Virginia is going out to a garden club once a month with Alicia. They have their small group of like-minded friends with whom they get together on a weekly basis. Virginia speaks with Alicia on the phone twice a day most days of the week. They do their morning call early as a check in, to make sure the other is well and safe. They then chat later in the day about the plans they make together if they don't end up at one or the other's house for coffee. This is a close friendship, and both one of these women will need to adjust if the other moves away or passes on.

DIETARY CONSIDERATION FOR VIRGINIA

The general recommendations for clients with congestive heart failure is to follow a heart healthy, sodium and fluid restricted diet. Given her reduced ejection fraction, total abstinence of alcohol would be encouraged. Given her ischemic heart disease and the need for stenting, in addition to her cholesterol-lowering medication, a heart healthy diet such as the Mediterranean diet would be a reasonable choice. Colourful fruits and vegetables with anti-oxidant natural ingredients, along with omega 3 fatty acid foods (fish) and limited red meat consumption, will all be reasonable choices. Her main goal is to improve her breathing and fitness level, and she's not currently interested in losing weight, so her Mediterranean diet with a healthy mix of macronutrients such as healthy fats, proteins, and whole grain carbohydrates, using the formula of 30kcal per kilogram of ideal body weight to maintain that weight, would suggest her daily intake be around 2200 kcal per day. Many computer and phone applications can help track her overall calories, sodium content and macronutrients of her diet if Virginia is motivated to track these items with her daily intake.

FINANCIAL CONSIDERATIONS FOR VIRGINIA

Virginia has some term life insurance (10-year term), purchased at age sixty-five when she was healthy, that is soon to expire. What are her options, and how does she plan for saving for possible personal care home institutionalization costs, if she ends up in long term care? Her insurance costs will go up within two years, and her "no evidence conversion options" will expire in two years. She has expressed a desire to leave a large amount of the life insurance benefit to a local non-profit animal rescue shelter. Given her poor health, a conversion option to permanent life insurance is possible and guarantees to last her lifetime. A term renewal will occur if she does nothing and will increase in price and only last until age eighty-five, when the policy expires. If her life expectancy is felt to be longer than ten years, the permanent insurance is her best option. If her cardiologist estimates her life expectancy to be significantly less than ten years, then term insurance may be acceptable. Of course, no one has the ability to predict the future, and even with the best planning, there is always some risk in life.[61] No matter which option she choses, the named beneficiary of the non-profit animal shelter will generate a tax-deductible donation for her terminal income tax return and will reduce her tax burden at death. As with all financial considerations as we age, this scenario needs to be fully explored with her certified financial planner.

ADVOCACY CONSIDERATIONS FOR VIRGINIA

Virginia has congestive heart failure with a reduced ejection fraction. While there are standards of medical therapy that now improve her quality and quantity of life, not every province makes it easy to get those medications. Because the lack of these medications can affect her quality and quantity of life, she has become a strong advocate for heart failure and regularly references the Canadian heart failure network. She follows the Heart and Stroke Foundation and advocates for preventative care to her other friends and acquaintances. There are many other areas of the country where new medications are released in a less restrictive manner than her own jurisdiction. She has been emailing and writing letters to her local MLA to advocate for the constituents, with the Ministry of Health on her behalf.

Virginia recognizes that she has a statistically lower chance of surviving a long time when compared to Alicia. She has made it clear to Alicia that should her condition deteriorate, she wishes to be palliated in her own bed at home. She has been seeking out how many palliative care beds there are in the community if she's unable to be managed safely at home. She is shocked by how little community

---

61 Please review with your own Certified Financial Planner.

support there is for palliative care. She has decided that she would like to try and advocate for improving this service, as she feels that it would be, in the end, a self-serving venture. She is planning on discussing her request for palliation with her primary care provider, should her circumstances worsen. Alicia has been declared a substitute decision maker on a representation agreement and Virginia will be meeting with her lawyer to review her will, her health care directives, and legalize that her best friend is to be medical and financial power of attorney, should she not be able to make decisions for her own care in future.

GENERAL HEALTH RECOMMENDATIONS FOR ALICIA

Alicia has had cancer and therefore needs to follow-up in a larger centre as recommended by her oncologist. Thus far, her cancer is in remission. She needs to continue with age-appropriate cancer screening as determined by her oncologist. Alicia doesn't have a primary care provider so gets her medications through the walk-in clinic. She is now diabetic and needs to have quarterly lab work and assessments done to review her glycemic control, kidney function, and blood pressure. She hasn't been walking 150 minutes per week at a target heart rate range for her age. Her inability to think forward into the future and social isolation may be signs that she is developing depression and should be screened for this with one of the many screening tools for depression (PHQ-9) at her next walk-in clinic visit. Alicia could even do an online assessment before her next visit to address her mood concerns, if she has the insight to recognize that a depression may be contributing to her symptoms. Her goal blood pressure should be less than 130/80 according to current guidelines. Her hemoglobin A1c should be under seven percent or lower, as long as she has no hypoglycemic events. She hasn't been told about getting her eyes examined every six to twelve months to rule out eye complications of her diabetes and hypertension. She does her own foot care but can't always see or reach to trim her toenails without nicking her skin. Nail care in diabetic should be done by a trained foot care nurse or podiatrist to avoid any possible open lesions that could lead to chronic diabetic foot ulcers or infections. Proper fitting shoes for walking (orthotics) may also help preserve the integrity of the skin of her feet and help facilitate proper exercise.

ACTIVITIES PLAN FOR ALICIA

Alicia can embark upon a standard exercise regimen (Activity Class C – see Chapter 8) like Maya or Deborah. The weight training and balance exercises can be completed on a daily basis. However, Alicia has had an artificial hip replacement, and she may not be able to do some of the strength training of the legs, such as squats or lunges. She would have to check with her orthopedic surgeon and/or physiotherapist about alternative exercises to improve her quadricep and hamstring strength. Being diabetic, Alicia should be sure to check her blood sugar before she starts any exercise. I would recommend that physically active diabetics take the opportunity to do continuous glucose monitoring for a month or two, so that they can see what their blood sugars do when they do their exercise programs. Continuous blood glucose monitoring will facilitate documentation of how different foods affect the blood sugars. She can easily correlate her sugars to any symptoms she might be experiencing. In the absence of a continuous glucose monitor, exercising in the morning after having a reasonable carbohydrate intake and holding off on oral medications until after exercise is done are both reasonable strategies to prevent low blood sugars with exercise. If diabetic clients require insulin, then a diabetic client should ideally know how much activity drops their blood sugar and can possibly take a slightly lower dose of short-acting insulin before the activity, or wait until after the activity to take the insulin once the post-exertion blood sugar is checked. All diabetics need to do their exercise regimen with both short-acting carbohydrates and fluids available in the event of hypoglycemia and dehydration. Items like dried cranberries or blueberries, short acting glucose tablets and other forms of quick acting sugars are easy to carry in a pocket. Additionally, diabetics should be wearing a medic alert bracelet when they are exercising outdoors or at a gym, in case hypoglycemia occurs suddenly and without warning.

BRAIN EXERCISES FOR ALICIA

Alicia needs to do whatever she can to increase her socialization and to improve overall cognitive function. She is computer savvy to a basic degree. She does play some computer games but doesn't do a lot of journaling, reading, writing, exercising, or interacting with neighbours. She enjoys her gardening when her yard is free of snow. Hopefully, she can go back to her garden club festivities now that the pandemic restrictions have lifted. She might need to have more focused Zoom interactions with her son, who lives further away. Weekly phone calls with her sons, to check in on how Alicia is doing, would be helpful. It may be necessary for both of her sons to keep separate tabs on their mother's overall well-being and for the sons to compare notes to ensure adequate socialization and overall safe functioning. Alicia likes music from her younger years. Perhaps encouraging listening to this comfort music along with exercising would be a start in helping her improve her cognition. Occasionally, an outside opinion from an allied health care professional, such as an occupational therapist, may provide some functioning insight that may be helpful in planning care for Alicia from afar. These professionals can do a cognitive screen in the comfort of the senior's own home and these assessments could offer invaluable insights in how the senior is really functioning. Recommendations regarding other available programs the senior may benefit from, could be suggested. There are more social prescribing programs that are being expanded that may be helpful for Alicia, if available in her community.

SOCIAL CONCERNS FOR ALICIA

In the wintertime, especially with the pandemic, there was very little social interaction. She was limited to getting her groceries and medications once every one or two weeks. She has a large yard and was overwhelmed by the amount of snow this past winter. Thankfully, she has neighbours who offered to snow blow her driveway and shovel for her, even before she made it outside. Alicia has not been doing a great deal of physical activity and the possibility of harming herself while shovelling or falling on ice remains a significant concern for her sons. While the neighbors were providing this service for free, Alicia needs to plan for and pay for yard/snow maintenance as an added winter expense. She is reluctant to leave her house despite having offers to live with one of her children, who lives far away. She isn't willing to downsize. She reluctantly does most of her own housework but had a housekeeper before the pandemic.

Family have noted that any new surroundings or changes in her normal pattern of activity causes a significant amount of anxiety and stress. Her sons are worried about her ability to drive any farther than the local grocery store or pharmacy. She's been feeling lonely, and all her activities in the past were put on hold because of the pandemic. She has only her friend, Virginia, who lives close by, but communicates with her other friends and siblings via email. She previously participated in an aqua fit program but hasn't re-joined the program due to the pandemic. She is no longer motivated to return to those previous programs.

She fell on a slippery deck in February while wearing only her slippers and pajamas. She hit her head and didn't tell her family members about it. She may benefit from a camera in her home or a life line/alert bracelet given her fall recently. The camera in her home has many privacy issues, so security options like this must be clearly discussed with her sons. She tells her two sons slightly different versions of stories when they individually see and speak with her. The sons have been comparing notes and noted that her ability to problem solve and think toward the future is quite impaired. They're worried about her ability to cope in her own home going forward. She has talked about going to an assisted living accommodation, transiently. She doesn't want to live with her oldest son, as she wouldn't be able to have her own things in his home. Because she doesn't have a primary care provider that knows her and her circumstances, Alicia is at ongoing risk of doing poorly in her home, increasing her risk of frailty, falls, and eventually institutionalization. At some point, the family may want to consider getting a private occupational therapist to do a cognitive screen and a home assessment for safety. Sometimes if a professional assesses and documents the safety challenges, the senior is more likely to follow the professional's advice over the family member's advice. The two sons could then have a conference with the health professional that performed the assessment to get a full report at the same time and asks questions together. Ideally, Alicia will have asked one of the sons to be her medical and financial power or attorney or substitute decision maker. If she has not done this with a lawyer, her sons will need to arrange for these important planning pieces to be completed.

DIETARY CONSIDERATION FOR ALICIA

Alicia has been losing weight since being diagnosed with diabetes and following a carbohydrate restricted diet, along with metformin. She has already lost twenty-five pounds and feels much better. In order to maintain her current weight, she would need to take 30 kcal per kilogram of ideal body weight that she wants to weigh. If she does increase her exercise regimen, those calories burned during the exercise program will need to be added back to that basic formula so that she is not in a catabolic state and burning more calories than she is consuming. Any heart healthy diet, Canada Food Guide, Mediterranean diet, or other low-salt, low saturated fat and carbohydrate restricted diet would acceptable to follow. If she had the desire, cognitive capacity, and motivation, seeing a dietitian and obtaining and following more detailed carbohydrate counting instructions might be suggested.

FINANCIAL CONSIDERATIONS FOR ALICIA

Alicia's house is paid for and she has no outstanding debts. Her car is paid for, although she drives a lot less than she used to. She has money in her tax-free savings account and has a pension. She follows a budget every year and makes adjustments as her needs change. Because she has two sons, one of which lives far away, she has purchased long-term care insurance in the event that she needs care in future, either in her home or in a facility. The details for accessing her long-term care insurance includes meeting criteria for a claim, waiting the appropriate pre determined waiting period for the insurance product, making the claim and proving that she requires assistance with at least two out of six activities of daily living, as stipulated in the insurance documents. Once the claim is processed and approved, the pre determined cash flow from the product comes to Alicia to pay for required care.

Given that Virginia and Alicia are good friends and live close together, they did initiate a discussion about pooling their resources and buying or building a suitable main floor level home with a shared kitchen but separated living spaces, bedroom, and bathrooms. They feel that by pooling their resources, each one of them would have money leftover to put toward care requirements in the future. How would this work?

This would be a much easier option if Virginia and Alicia were a common law or married couple. If they planned early enough, they could buy two separate life insurance policies to look after one another if either should pass away. Their wills need to stipulate leaving the home to the remaining partner.

As friends, this is more complicated. Both women and their families need to know what to expect when either one of the ladies passes away. It might be better for one woman to purchase the home with only her name on the title. The other could rent her share of space with a standard rental/lease agreement with some added details from a cohabitation perspective. The renter will need to relocate if the owner passes away and leaves the home to her beneficiaries. The owner could use the rent money to add to her savings for future care purposes. The assets of the home of the renter can be used to be put into a financial vehicle such as an accumulation annuity. There will be automatic withdrawals to cover the accommodation and living costs. The automatic withdrawals can be adjusted according to account details.[62] If the renter passes away, the remaining funds in the accumulation annuity bypass probate and go directly to the named beneficiaries. Please consult with your own financial team before considering any of these suggestions.

---

62 Contact your certified financial planner for options

ADVOCACY CONSIDERATIONS FOR ALICIA

Alicia likely has the start of dementia or cognitive decline.[63] Social isolation may accelerate this, and because Alicia doesn't have a live-in partner, she's at risk for further decline without interventions. Her family will need to seek out programs that Alicia might consider, such as a geriatric day hospital. The sons may need to go with Alicia to a doctor's appointment to ask for a referral to a geriatrician to initiate a comprehensive geriatric assessment. The sons need to be more involved with Alicia and her daily interactions, as she has already fallen once and didn't have the insight to recognize the hazard of the fall, and did not have the judgment of being aware that this type of event should be reported to her family or primary care provider.

REFLECTION AND DISCUSSION

Virginia and Alicia are great friends and rely on each other for their day-to-day safety check ins. Together, they each provide socialization and brain exercises for one another, but they have complicated physical conditions and exercise/activity strategies are different for each woman. This scenario illustrates that a "one size fits all strategy" for seniors does not work when prescribing exercise or activity programs. Every senior will require an individualized strategy for providing advice in the domains of general health, activity prescriptions, social prescriptions and financial considerations. Aging is complicated and every senior needs many team members to provide the best options for individuals while keeping the seniors personal goals as the driving focus of any plan.

---

63 "A Dementia Strategy for Canada: Together We Aspire," Government of Canada, accessed August 24, 2022, https://www.canada.ca/en/public-health/services/publications/diseases-conditions/dementia-strategy.html.

CHAPTER 12:
PREPARATION FOR ACTION
IN THE EIGHTIES

There is a fountain of youth: it is your mind, your talents, the creativity you bring to your life and the lives of people you love. When you learn to tap this source, you will truly have defeated age. —Sophia Loren

Clinical Scenario:

Karl is eighty-seven years old and a retired railroad worker. He is cognitively very sharp but physically has issues with mobility, urinary incontinence, and fecal incontinence. He has diabetes, peripheral neuropathy from diabetes, hypertension, dyslipidemia, frailty, abdominal aortic aneurysm, and spinal stenosis. Chronic leg swelling further impairs his mobility, and he needs to use a two-wheeled walker.

GENERAL HEALTH
RECOMMENDATIONS FOR KARL

Karl has outlived the average life expectancy for a man. While he should likely be congratulated on this feat, he has mentioned on numerous times that he is totally shocked that he made it to this age! And still, he keeps on going. He is not, and has never been, the epitome of health. To his, and his family's surprise, his medical conditions are under reasonable control. He has been denied surgery for his spinal stenosis due to his age and complex medical conditions. He quit smoking five years ago and could be referred for a low dose CT scan of the thorax, but finding a lung cancer at this age would not change his opinion on therapy. He has lived a good life and has expectations of passing within the next few years. He does not want to pursue any life-prolonging surgeries or treatments. If his abdominal aneurysm suddenly increases in size, he is aware that it might rupture and his life would be over quite quickly. He continues to go for yearly assessments with an ultrasound of the aorta, so that he can be mentally prepared for a change in status. His aneurysm was detected by his primary care provider as part of a once in a life time screening event for abdominal aneurysms. Karl has been a non-drinker for thirty years. He hasn't had any issues with his liver in the past, considering that in his youth he was a drinker. Karl is at risk for a stroke and takes a low dose of daily aspirin. He hasn't had any stroke-like symptoms but does not wish to know whether the blood flow to the brain is impaired. He has been offered an ultrasound of his carotid arteries to assess for that, but he has declined. He has a higher than acceptable blood sugar level for his age, and is aware that hypoglycemic events would be detrimental to his brain. He has an advanced care plan posted on the fridge of his assisted living apartment that denotes a "do not resuscitate" status. His family is aware of his wishes. A younger version of Karl, especially one who did not have a primary care provider, may also have benefitted from an annual self review of a men's general health checklist.[64]

ACTIVITIES PLAN FOR KARL

Karl is unsteady and not able to walk safely without a walker, primarily due to his spinal stenosis, but also because he has diabetic neuropathy and no sensation from his shins down to his toes on both legs. From an exercise perspective, Karl can certainly do any sitting, stretch, and strengthening classes, three to five times per week, and he can embark upon light weight training of his upper body. He would be advised to start with an activity Class A plan as set out in Chapter 8. If going to a gym to exercise, it may be safer for him to use weight machines, rather than free weights, to avoid dropping any weight and injuring a diabetic foot. His legs are weak but there are overriding neuromuscular conditions present that make improvement of leg strength and functionality likely impossible. As he will rely more and more on the strength of his arms, I would encourage practising repetitively lifting his bottom up from the chair and holding the pose for as long as he can. This can increase his arm and shoulder strength. Because Karl is considered unsteady and unsafe without his walker, Karl could try

---

64 Men's Health Checklist - Made for Canadian Men (menshealthfoundation.ca)

the balance exercises as outlined in Chapter 7, but would have to have a strong chaperone or work out buddy nearby, in case he lost his balance and fell. He would also need to have the ability to grab on to the sink or a safety bar if balance starts to fail. Overall, there would be more risk and less benefit to balance exercises in Karl's situation. When Karl is sitting in a supportive chair, he may attempt to do straight leg raising, eight to twelve repetitions per leg, and bent leg raising, eight to twelve repetitions per leg. He can work up to three sets of repetitions every second day. From a leg mobility perspective, I would recommend that Karl use a mini exercise bike, if available, that he can ride from the safety of his favourite couch or chair. These minibikes can be extremely helpful with all the computer meetings that individuals have had to do virtually, since the pandemic started. If I'm in a meeting or conference, I continuously ride this quiet machine for as long as possible. While I don't really get my heart rate into the target heart rate zone, I'm definitely exercising my legs and burning some calories instead of just sitting on my behind.

BRAIN EXERCISES FOR KARL

Karl has been a carpenter all his life. He has the ability to look at things on two-dimensional paper and figure out how to make them three-dimensional and beautiful. He no longer practises those skills due to his physical deterioration. He has a grade ten education. He did very well as a senior shop foreman in the railway industry prior to retirement. He continues to be an avid gardener, growing tomatoes and cucumbers on his patio in the summertime. He keeps some houseplants in his assisted living suite during the winter. He is a fan of sports and old movies. He does word search and crossword puzzles on a daily basis. He plays old-fashioned solitaire with a deck of cards by himself. He's still able to manage his personal finances, although his daughters have already been established as a dual power of attorneys. Karl continues to do a variety of brain exercises that are listed in Chapter 7. He is not interested in exploring new projects as he gets a great deal of joy from his current routine. His daughters note that his cognitive function is still very good for his age and agree that pushing him to do more brain activities, would likely not yield any significant added benefit.

SOCIAL CONCERNS FOR KARL

Since Karl moved into his assisted living suite three years ago, he has become quite the social butterfly. He has many female friends in the home that he went to grade school with, and has some male friends in the residence with whom he plays pool on a weekly basis. He's a very social creature and likes to have coffee and engage in current events discussions with his fellow residents in the home. He speaks English and used to speak both Polish and Ukrainian, but since his mother passed away twenty-five years ago, and he has no siblings, his birth languages are no longer present. If he had no daughters or other family members to look after him, Karl would be considered to be a "kinless senior."[65]

Kinless seniors are becoming an increasingly vulnerable group of seniors where social isolation and lonely living conditions can contribute to premature death and decreased quality of life.

Karl's only significant social concern is that the pandemic lockdowns resulted in the enforcement of a lot of "rules" in the residence that he did not appreciate. He felt penalized with the lockdowns, especially when he couldn't eat his meals in the dining room with his friends and neighbours. In these early, post pandemic months, his biggest issue is that he has the desire to travel (anywhere for a brief vacation), but his physical condition makes most travel choices unrealistic and unattainable options. One of his daughters lives out of the country for six months of the year, so this limits his family outings during this time. When his oldest child is available, there will be many social outings with children, grandchildren, and great-grandchildren during these months. Of course, social events with young children do make one predisposed to a variety of viral illnesses when families are together. Karl is aware of these risks but chooses to participate in family events and is realistic, but unafraid of potential illness consequences.

---

65 https://www-nytimes-com.cdn.ampproject.org/c/s/www.nytimes.com/2022/12/03/
    health/elderly-living-alone.amp.html

There has been no cognitive decline, and Karl appears to be keeping his brain as active as it can be. Karl continues to drive a vehicle, and one of his daughters has been in the vehicle, with him driving. She has noted that he's going through the majority of quieter side streets and avoiding big intersections. His stop time still seems adequate, as his usual rate of speed is slightly below the posted speed limit. Given his peripheral neuropathy and spinal stenosis, his daughter is aware that he will soon not be able to drive safely. Currently, Karl uses his vehicle to "escape" the assisted living building when he's bored, needing medications or groceries, or just wanting to get out of the residence. His safe driving ability will be an issue that needs to be addressed within the next six to twelve months. He has a plan for selling his vehicle to his grandson when that time comes. His assisted living residence has a senior's van and regularly takes the residents to appointments regularly so arranging travel in the future is not a concern.

DIETARY CONSIDERATIONS FOR KARL

Karl is a long-standing diabetic who is on insulin and metformin. His goal should be to maintain his weight without weight loss or weight gain, as his BMI is 29. Avoiding hypoglycemia should be the key focus, as he already has end organ damage from his diabetes (neuropathy), but hypoglycemic events would be detrimental to his cognitive health. He is sitting with a hemoglobin A1c of 8.5 percent, which is reasonable given his age and the need for preventing hypoglycemia. If he was twenty years younger, clinicians would advise for him to have a much lower target for hemoglobin A1c. A diabetic diet is offered at his assisted living residence and more stringent carbohydrate control, although may be beneficial, is not an option for this gentleman. He has made it very clear to his family that after having diabetes for thirty years and approaching ninety, he is not interested in making any changes to his diet.

FINANCIAL CONSIDERATIONS FOR KARL

Karl grew up in an era where he didn't actively invest or trust market-based funds. He always felt that it was a significant risk, and while he does have a pension from the railroad, he chose to sell his home and put that money into an accumulation annuity to augment his income. The details of the accumulation annuity are as follows: This is a non-registered account, which means that all interest is taxable as income, and as a non registered account, upon death, all funds remaining will bypass probate and go to his named beneficiaries. Beneficiaries will receive funds once a death certificate is received after the claim is made and processed.

Karl has prepaid for his funeral costs, or at least eighty percent in current dollar value. His bank accounts have both daughters as power of attorney with signing authority so that when he passes, they can pay for the rest of the funeral costs without the bank accounts being frozen.

Probate is the "death tax." No one wants to call it that, but when one dies, the government does take its share of remaining funds. This varies from province to province. Your certified financial planner will have numerous strategies to reduce probate at the time of death, but this requires *extensive* early financial planning, which needs to start earlier if you have large assets, debt, or a complicated estate. Ideally this should be looked at before the age of eighty, but there is really never an issue with planning too soon.

Karl has no personal life insurance but will have enough money to pay his expenses, with his pension combined with his proceeds invested from the sale of his home. This money is expected to last to age one hundred, unless the need for more personal care changes, which will deplete his resources faster.

Karl has been gifting money to his children. This is a good strategy for avoiding probate as long there is enough to pay his expenses. He also has an emergency fund in his bank account of $20,000 as a safe buffer in case circumstances change.

PROBATE ESTIMATES ACROSS CANADA (2020 VALUES)

PROVINCE	VALUE OF ESTATE	FEES/TAXES
ALBERTA	>$250,000	**MAXIMUM** $525
BRITISH COLUMBIA	>$50,000	**MAXIMUM** $350 + 1.4%
MANITOBA	>$10,000	**MAXIMUM** $ 70 + 0.7%
NEW BRUNSWICK	>$20,000	**MAXIMUM** 0.5%
NEWFOUNDLAND	>$1000	**MAXIMUM** $60 + 0.6%
NWT	>$250,000	**MAXIMUM** $435
NOVA SCOTIA	>$100,000	**MAXIMUM** $1002.65 + 1.695%
NUNAVIT	>$250,000	**MAXIMUM** $400
ONTARIO	>$50,000	**MAXIMUM** $250 + 1.5%
PEI	>$100,000	**MAXIMUM** $400 + 0.4%
QUEBEC	DEPENDS ON WILL	**REFER TO LOCAL GOVERNMENT**
SASK	ANY	**MAXIMUM** 0.7%
YUKON	>$25,000	**MAXIMUM** $140

ADVOCACY CONSIDERATIONS FOR KARL

Karl is still able to advocate for himself. He's a very vocal member in his assisted living complex and has written numerous letters to the administrators of his retirement community home. He absolutely understands the legitimacy of the restrictions during the pandemic but felt the need to advocate for his fellow residents with their concerns. While he realized he was in a very high-risk category for COVID-19 complications, he was not happy with the forced social isolation. He was compliant with his immunizations and booster shots for COVID-19. Other than experiencing a very long winter indoors, Karl doesn't believe that he needs to change his living arrangements and he still enjoys his choice to move into an assisted living residence. He continues to advocate for himself and other residents, and his letters written to the residence managers, make sense, are concise and well written. This advocacy for his group of friends and neighbours should be encouraged.

REFLECTION AND DISCUSSION

This chapter reflects the everchanging landscape of health care, accommodation, travel, and financial needs of seniors, as age advances. There is the constant requirement of adjusting plans for the elderly as the goals of the individual take precedent over trying to make the individual comply with recommended health directives. Karl's scenario reflects the need for seniors to control their own destiny, as much as possible and encouraging this advocacy promotes quality of life and a sense of purpose in many of these senior advocates. It is so important for all individuals to be heard, especially when living in outside of their own home. Fostering independence and helping them be heard should be the goal of every interaction with these valuable and knowledgeable senior members of society!

CHAPTER 13:
PREPARATION FOR ACTION AT NINETY-PLUS YEARS

Don't let the expectations and opinions of other people affect your decisions. It's your life, not theirs. Do what matters most to you; do what makes you feel alive and happy. Don't let the expectations and ideas of others limit who you are. If you let others tell you who you are, you are living their reality—not yours. There is more to life than pleasing people. There is much more to life than following others' prescribed path. There is so much more to life than what you experience right now. You need to decide who you are for yourself. Become a whole being. Adventure.
—Roy T. Bennett

Clinical scenario:

Methuselah is ninety-three years old. He is on cholesterol medication, blood pressure medication, and aspirin after having a remote transient ischemic attack (mini stroke) years ago. Up until six months ago, he was snow blowing his and the neighbour's driveways and used a ride-on lawn mower to do many of the neighbours' front lawns. He was active in his shop and able to fix almost everything. He developed unusual growths on his legs that were diagnosed to be a connective tissue cancer. He did not want a leg amputation and decided to proceed with extensive surgery, with muscle and skin grafting in order to prevent the tumors from growing and eventually breaking through the skin. He then required five weeks of radiation therapy.

GENERAL HEALTH RECOMMENDATIONS FOR METHUSELAH

Methuselah is a nonagenarian that went from a robust physiological status to very frail. While he has already outlived the standard life expectancy for a North American man, he needs to focus on preventing falls, fractures, and hospitalization. He has already made the decision that he would never want to go into a long-term care home. This was the primary reason for refusing to consider a leg amputation that may have been curative for his cancer. He has already survived prostate cancer. This new cancer has resulted in the complicating factor of having chronic pain. Methuselah is on narcotics for pain management. He is often confused and sleepy and doesn't always remember when friends or neighbours come to visit. He needs to focus on being safe within his home. In his medicated state, he should not be attempting to go down to his basement at all. As his shower is located in the basement, he might need assistance when showering. Methuselah lives alone and his "lady friend" brings him a hot meal every evening for dinner. But this friend is not willing or physically able to assist with activities of daily living such as bathing or dressing. Methuselah is at risk for falls. When changing positions, he needs to slowly get up from the lying to sitting position first. Then once he is certain that he is not dizzy, he can stand up and walk with his required walking aid, such as a cane or walker. Methuselah has never considered himself to be "old." Prior to his cancer diagnosis and surgery, he was very good at general machine maintenance, fixing small engines, and had the ability to problem solve almost any issue that developed in his day-to-day life. Since his surgery, there has been a marked deterioration in his physical and mental capabilities. He is not felt to be safe at home and has been instructed not to drive while his leg heals. His narcotic use, which is necessary for pain control, renders him forgetful, sleepy, and teary. Methuselah has constant reminders that his body condition has changed and that he needs to be more cautious in order to avoid dizziness, instability, and falls.

There are no other general health recommendations for Methuselah with regards to illness prevention or screening other than the falls prevention as outlined above. The need for home care support in Methuselah's own home is critical for the next several weeks or months. Methuselah has reluctantly agreed to have home care assistant attend to him for the next few weeks until he recovers more function.

If his condition deteriorates, the goals of care should focus on comfort and quality of life for his remaining days. Methuselah was frail after his surgery and before the radiation but has become frailer since the radiation therapy. He has felt fatigued every day, and for the last month, he's unable to walk more than fifteen feet or climb a flight of stairs. He now has numerous comorbid conditions of cancer, hypertension, arthritis, mild stroke, and he has lost more than five percent of his body weight over the last six months. His FRAIL score is 5/5 and the prognosis is guarded. Palliative care would be the next most appropriate step to consider unless he has a miraculous turnaround within the next few weeks or months.

ACTIVITIES PLAN FOR METHUSELAH

Methuselah is in the recovery phase of an acute surgical intervention with subsequent radiation therapy. He is walking within his home ten to fifteen feet with a two-wheeled walker or a cane. He has a lot of pain and is taking narcotics for the pain in his bones. His skin grafting hasn't healed well with the radiation therapy, and he requires homecare to dressings on his wounds several times a week. He needs assistance with his basic activities of daily living including bathing, meal preparation, and dressing. At this point in time, he is not able to do any exercise regimen, as his affected leg needs to be elevated during the day. Methuselah could do a light weight regimen with either low weight dumbbells or resistance tubing to work his arms, both biceps and triceps. When he's in an armchair, he can lift his butt off the chair by using his arms and holding it for a few seconds to increase the strength of his upper body. He would not be a candidate for balance exercises until such time that:

1. his leg has completely healed
2. he can walk without a walking aid
3. he has no *significant* pain
4. he has been weaned of his narcotic pain medications

Methuselah doesn't have family nearby, so it's important that he has the opportunity for social interaction through phone calls, homecare, or visits from friends/family/neighbours.

DIETARY CONSIDERATIONS

At this point, he will need adequate protein intake to enhance his healing. He may have diminished appetite due to constipation from his narcotics, and he will require regular fiber, adequate fluid intake, and possibly laxatives to keep his bowels moving every day. His lady friend brings him an evening meal and home care supports assist with meal preparation at breakfast and lunch. If inadequate calories or nutrients are taken in during the day, protein supplements may offer some enhanced nutrition if tolerated by Methuselah.

Methuselah is in the recovery phase of two massive body insults in the last four months. He has had extensive surgery, followed by immobility while healing, and then radiation therapy. These are all catabolic processes and weight loss and muscle wasting has occurred. He hasn't been consuming a great deal of protein due to the recent cost of meat secondary to inflation. He has never used any supplemental protein powder and doesn't like the taste of protein drinks. His appetite seems to be improving on a daily basis, but his overall caloric and protein intake are low. His body weight is currently 80 kg, and he was 85 kg prior to the surgery and radiation. He's a tall man, and we'd like to get him back up to the 85 kg. If he uses a formula for weight gain requiring 40 kcal per kilo of ideal body weight, he would need to consume 3400 kcal a day and take in about 80–85 grams of protein per day to facilitate wound healing and increase overall muscle strength. There are a variety of both plant-based and whey protein-based supplements. Some protein powders are tasteless and dissolve in any fluid. These products can be added to one's morning cup of coffee and there is no change in taste or consistency of the coffee. The average amount of protein per scoop varies between 10–30 grams. It wouldn't matter what kind of protein supplement one chooses, as long as it is palatable and affordable.

Other ways to increase protein intake would include increasing portion sizes of meat, eggs, and meat alternative products such as tofu or tempeh. Adding soft tofu to a milkshake will also increase the protein content. Making a cooked custard sauce using eggs and high fat milk and then cooled appropriately in the fridge and used within forty-eight hours is an option. The custard sauce can also be added to desserts and, if unsweetened, cream soups. If his cancer isn't cured, one could expect that Methuselah will continue to be in a catabolic process and continue to lose weight despite all best efforts. If this is the case, readjusting goals of care and focusing on improved quality of life would be appropriate at this time. Further lifestyle and nutritional information are available from the BC government website www.to.gov.bc.ca under "BC Seniors Guide." A number in this part of the website for a registered dietitian through the HealthLinkBC portal by calling 8–1–1 or by going to their website and entering "contact a dietitian" in the search.

BRAIN EXERCISES FOR METHUSELAH

With the narcotic use, it will be very easy for him to become drowsy or delirious if he's over medicated. His girlfriend and home care workers will need to assess his mentation and decision making on a regular basis. If he enjoys activities such as playing cards or other table games, this should be encouraged when interest and energy allow. At this point in time, Methuselah will need to focus on quality of life. Methuselah has stopped driving due to his narcotic use which is appropriate given his current condition. Once his narcotic use has diminished, further brain exercises can be considered in future.

SOCIAL CONCERNS FOR METHUSELAH

Methuselah is at high risk for social isolation, and any opportunity to get him safely out of his home to have visits with friends or family should be offered. He is at high risk for elder abuse from a financial position, as the narcotics, which he requires for pain, impair his decision making. His powers of attorney may need to review the banking situation and ensure there are no unusual purchases or withdrawals. The family will need to take over financial affairs at some point in time. There was a significant number of neighbours coming by to "check in" on Methuselah. While most of these individuals have very good intentions, the sudden presence of a "new friend" should alert the home care workers of the potential for elder abuse, especially if Methuselah has not had a pre-existing relationship with this individual in the past. Seniors with severe illness, cognitive decline, or incapacity due to medications are at high risk for elder abuse.

FINANCIAL CONSIDERATIONS FOR METHUSELAH

From a financial perspective, given his change in overall health status, Methuselah and his family may want to have a preliminary meeting with a financial planner to discuss executor duties and administration of the estate, probate, and tax implications at the time of death.

What if Methuselah wants to leave money to his girlfriend, and his sons are not in agreement? While Methuselah is still competent and directing his finances, Methuselah can gift his girlfriend at any point in time. He has made specifications in his will to bequeath some of his assets to her upon his death. The will is legal and binding and is recent. Although the sons could challenge the will, it would be costly and, quite frankly, a waste of time and money, and *all assets* would be frozen until settled. Then probate must be cleared. It could take years for his estate to settle if legal action were to occur.

What if both sons, who have power of attorney and banking privileges, decide to sell Methuselah's house without his permission? At this point, with signing authority/POA already done, the sons could take these steps without Methuselah's permission. This is a risk when giving POAs signature capabilities. Once the POAs have been enacted (documentation required to let financial institutions know that POA is decision maker), then all instructions will now come from the POA. If Methuselah works with a certified financial planner, he may have designated a "Trusted Contact Person."[66] This is a person designated by the client who can serve as intermediary to help prevent unknown financial abuses from continuing. If there are suspicious activities with the client's investments, this Trusted Person can liaise with the client to facilitate exploration of unusual activities. This Trusted Person has

---

66 See Client Reforms from the Financial Industry Regulators (https://www.facsc.ca as an example)

been authorized to communicate with the client and help explore the rationale of activity and is a safeguard against elder financial abuse. If the certified financial planner suspects financial abuse, he/she is required to report the concerns to the regulatory body for "account investigation," possibly pausing all transactions until clarified. If Methuselah is cognitively still able to direct financial activities, then he may need to seek legal counsel to revoke the POAs and meet with the bank to undo the signatories on the accounts.

Methuselah does not have his funeral paid for, but his sons currently can access his banking funds to pay for the end-of-life costs.

How can Methuselah avoid probate with his estate? He has already placed his sons on title, which will decrease the estate value. All registered investments that have named beneficiaries (funds will go to the sons) would still be subject to Canada Revenue Agency terminal tax return rules for "fully redeemed" as income in the terminal tax return of Methuselah. Gifting money to his family or friends before death will decrease the impact of probate.

ADVOCACY CONSIDERATIONS FOR METHUSELAH

This scenario illustrates how one individual can go from being very robust to extremely frail within a very short time frame. The most important things to do at this stage of life are to adequately review and document goals of care, as it has been shown that frailty is a marker for both poor outcomes in the ICU setting as well as neurologic recovery after a resuscitation attempt with CPR. While the patient is competent, he will need to be certain that his final will and testament is in order, he has dealt with his home and dispersion of assets, he has both legal and enduring medical power of attorney to make medical decisions on his behalf, and that family is present when he discusses his goals of care, including resuscitation status. While still competent, he could even entertain the concept of medical assistance in dying (MAID).[67]

---

67 https://www.canada.ca/en/health-canada/services/medical-assistance-dying.html

REFLECTION AND DISCUSSION

Unlike the biblical Methuselah, this man will not survive to age 969 years. It's likely that by the time this book is published, he will have passed away. In the end, hopefully this Methuselah will reflect on his life and be settled with the decisions he has made as he approaches the end of this journey. If you know a Methuselah, these are exceptional individuals with skills, knowledge, and memories that can only be appreciated by interacting regularly with them. If you take the time to listen to these elders, your own life will be enhanced. We can't avoid death, but we all want to be in control of our circumstances until that point, when the grim reaper eventually comes knocking.

CHAPTER 14:
ESSENTIALS OF HOME ASSESSMENT AND ALLIED HEALTH PROFESSIONAL INPUT

Safety isn't expensive, it's price less. —Anonymous

The last chapter is focused on the possibility of requiring health professional in one's home to assist with care, when it is required. As a caregiver, there is nothing like a home visit. I am privileged to be invited into a client's home for a home assessment or palliative care visit. Home visits are not realistically available in everyday practice in every community. When there are opportunities that the clinician can do a home visit or tag along with an allied health professional as they do a home functionality/safety assessment, it is very enlightening and rewarding. While an occupational assessment is part of the more comprehensive geriatric assessment, these objective assessments regarding the functionality of the accommodations/living situations are instrumental in determining possible solutions to any dysfunctional issue in the home. They are requested on behalf of the client, family or health care team, to review the functional and safety concerns in a client's own home. These assessments can determine if the patient has any functional unmet needs. This could include items such as mobility assistant devices, that can facilitate independent functioning and ultimately improve the quality of life of the client, while continuing to reside in the comfort of one's own home.

The assessment of functional status is critical when looking at how anyone manages in their own home. There are normal aging processes that are complicated by acute and chronic illnesses and these conditions, when they flare, may result in hospitalization. This can then contribute to an often, step wise decline in functional status, with each hospitalization. Hospital-associated deconditioning occurs when patients become ill, require intravenous therapies, are generally weakened by the acute component of the condition, spend a great deal of time in bed, and sometimes, receive medications that further contribute to developing weakness. The weakened status worsens with each day the patient is in hospital or immobilized. The hospital stay can impact the client to such a degree, that they may not be able to live independently in the community following their hospital stay. This need for a change in living environment may be transient, but often, it results in a long-term change in living arrangements. Most patients are not ready for this to happen when they are admitted with an illness felt to be transient. A functional assessment, which is done in hospital by both occupational and physiotherapists (OT and PT), will allow hospitals to make decisions on the feasibility of a safe hospital discharge. A safe hospital discharge involves the patient going home to a supportive environment, with the required care/services already present and results in no medication errors, an improvement in functional status and no untoward events. Safe hospital discharges result in a lower hospital readmission rate. In my own family, there are elderly members who function very well in their own home with their own routine and when there are no disruptions to the daily schedule. However, these same individuals, when they are removed from their home environment, and join family for an extended visit or vacation, are unable to safely function without direction. It is often in this scenario, when objective deficiencies in their ability to problem solve and cope, are unearthed.

A functional home assessment, either before a hospitalization or as part of a pre-discharge planning exercise, can provide crucial objective data, to assist with planning recovery and rehabilitation needs. Such needs could include homemaker services, meal preparation, personal or nursing care, and general supervision. The activities of daily living (ADLs) are the basic self-care tasks and skills we need to look after ourselves, and these are usually developed in early childhood. The instrumental activities of daily living (iADLs) are the more complex skills that allow an individual to manage at home and be fully independent. Deficits in these combined activities often correspond with the type and amount of assistance that will be required. If the care requirements needed to remain safely in the home are excessive (that is beyond what the local home support community services can provide), our current societal and health care standard is to initiate registration for long-term care placement.

During in-home assessments, the allied health professionals will review the client's ability to walk in and around the home and outside on short walks. This assessment includes the ability to climb and descend stairs, ability to perform independent ADLs and the professional will formulate an overall opinion with regards to the safe ability to function at home or "age in place."[68] Discussions from one of the team members regarding nutrition concerns, which can range from acquiring groceries to making meals to ultimately getting the required nutrition into the client safely and without choking is critical. The home assessment may also include dressing and grooming (cognitively appropriate selection of weather-appropriate clothes and footwear, the ability to physically dress oneself, and managing one's personal grooming and appearances). Toileting is assessed by observing how an individual gets to and from the toilet, uses the toilet facilities appropriately, and includes the functional ability to clean oneself after using the toilet. Newer luxury items like bidet type toilet seats may prove beneficial in some of these functions. Self care and bathing observations assess how safely an individual can function in the bathtub or shower, as this is a high-risk area for falls. Mobility assessments also include transferring from one position to the other (in bed or chair) and being able to move within the home from bed to chair or to wheelchair, standing in order to grasp a walker or other assistive devices and stability when standing that helps determine safe functional status.

The iADLs are more the organizational and cognitive skills that allow us to manage finances, arrange transportation, perform shopping and meal preparation, achieve housekeeping and home maintenance tasks, communicate via telephone, mail or other technological devices (computer, email and text), and safe management of medications. This includes obtaining medications and compliance with taking medications. In the comprehensive geriatric toolkit, which is available to caregivers providing geriatric care services, there are many scoring

---

68 www.seniorliving.org/aging-in-place/

systems or indices that the care provider can use. Some of these include names like the Barthel index (which includes written, modified and online versions), the Bristol ADL scale and other cognitive screening tools that are too numerous to mention. The important point about these tools for the client and their family members, is that the majority of the tools utilized by the team, have been tested in large populations and assist the team in organizing care that would promote the safest plan, that gives the senior, the best chance to age in place safely.

In my family, having these professionals come into the home environment, who are not known to the client or family, may be perceived as being intrusive. However, clients and families need to be assured that everyone's collective goal on the health-care team, is to keep elderly people functioning safely and as independently in their home, for as long as possible. But clients, families and care givers all need to be realistic about the expectations of existing safely and independently as one ages! The health care team is not out to "put you in a home." All healthcare professionals believe that home is best, but only if you're able to manage safely without the risk of harm coming to the individual, who is often living alone. If an individual's goal is to be alone and independent, and it's not safe, then either home is not the best place for you or home alone and without assistance is no longer in one's best interest. All individuals experiencing these truths about the inability to function safe, alone, in their own home, have options. The challenge for the client, family, and team is to explore all feasible and realistic options and then assist the client in making the best decision for the individual at the time, keeping in mind the client's goals in the short and long term. What matters most to the client should direct all further care decisions.

CHAPTER SUMMARY

As I stated at the beginning of the chapter, I value the privilege and have been honoured to be a part of any home visit, when it occurs. There is such valuable information obtained by watching people function in their own home. When it comes time for your family member or you to have a home assessment, note that everyone, from your family members to the health-care team, want what is best for you.

This chapter offered a basic overview of the concepts and purpose of home assessments and why these reviews are instrumental in planning a safe client discharge from hospital or an outpatient assessment to determine continued feasibility to continue living at home independently. I would urge readers to embrace any home visit that is offered, as the collective goal of the team is for all seniors to safely "age in place."

CHAPTER 15:
NEED/ROLE FOR COMPREHENSIVE GERIATRIC ASSESSMENTS

Aging is an extraordinary process where you become the person you always should've been. —David Bowie

As a modern Western society, younger generations have not always valued the elderly. As our aging population demographic will increase substantially over the next twenty-five years, all members of society are respectfully asked to consider the human rights of all ages, races, and religions in our world. The United Nations has an excellent resource for reviewing literature and initiating discussions regarding the human rights of the seniors' populations.[69] As a late middle-aged adult at the end of the baby boomer generation, I have perceived some degree of age discrimination in the workplace. I am fearful for ongoing stigmatization, stereotyping, and marginalization as I age. One of my acquaintances is particularly aware of his diagnosis of early dementia and has expressed concerns that phone calls with his children often result in him feeling that he is a burden. He perceives his children to be very impatient with him. This is not an isolated incident. The Public Health Agency of Canada has been advertising for the general public to be kind, patient, and understanding if we expect that an individual has some cognitive impairment.[70]

As I mentioned in an earlier chapter, our population is aging and there is a paucity of geriatric specialists in our country. This means that only the most critically impaired seniors in society are accessing these specialists. Access to this health care service will mean that at some point in time, a comprehensive geriatric assessment (CGA) will be done. While this is excellent for those individuals who receive

---

69 OHCHR | About the human rights of older persons

70 "A Dementia Strategy for Canada: Together We Aspire," Government of Canada, accessed August 24, 2022, https://www.canada.ca/en/public-health/services/publications/diseases-conditions/dementia-strategy.html.

this specialized care, there are many more marginally functioning frail elders in the community that do not have access to any of these services. In addition, many elderly clients in my local area do not even have access to primary health care. This gap is widening daily and we, as a society, are in for troubling times ahead. And while the gap between the lack geriatricians and an increase in older population increases, this puts more pressure on primary care providers and specialists to provide more enhanced geriatric care in their daily practice. This happens at a time when primary health care and community specialist availability is at an all time low across the country. What are the options for our collective communities? This is a disturbing realization. By writing this book, it is my intention to rally our communities to take notice of our reality in health care. Can an individual do anything to improve our access to primary care, geriatric care, specialist care and hospital care? I have some hope that this will occur in the near future. Hopefully, having read this book, you will feel educated, empowered, and prepared to take on the challenges that lie ahead for all of us.

For now, we need to rely on our families, friends, neighbours, pharmacists, and health care providers to help us objectively take notice when one is not functioning well in society or at home. How do concerned individuals proceed with getting help for a family member, friend, colleague or acquaintance in these complicated times?

This is such a tall task.

I would suggest the first order of business is to initiate a conversation about the concerns with the individual him/herself. One can explore the concerns in a non threatening manner. Concerned individuals can provide reading materials or discuss available programs. Friends can ask permission from the senior to have a conversation with family members to discuss any concerns. The senior in question needs to guide the assistance, if and when, it is desired. If the senior is willing to seek out assistance, then programs at the municipal, provincial and federal governments are available. Sometimes, an older adult needs assistance to navigate the new reality of online access to services. Local volunteer groups that assist seniors can be contacted, if agreeable by the older adult of concern. Having frank conversation about frailty, falling and memory on a regular basis as a "check in" with a group of friends also seems non threatening and viable. However, at every point in a discussion, the senior must be absolutely comfortable with proceeding with conversations, assessments, and care plans.

What might be some of the circumstances that could trigger the need for a comprehensive geriatric assessment? Certainly, repeated emergency room visits, accidents, falls, injuries, deterioration of chronic health conditions, and an overall appearance of lack of nutrition or hygiene should prompt a discussion, sooner rather than later. I believe that society needs to work together as a larger "community" to improve elder care across the entire country. This certainly has tax payer and political implications at all levels of politics.

SEXUALLY ACTIVE SENIORS

There will be a time in many of our lives, when we might need to have a formal comprehensive geriatric assessment done by a geriatric team. This can be a blessing. It's a general overview of how physical, cognitive, emotional, spiritual, and sexual needs can be met. When I was a very young physician, I was absolutely astounded at the number of older adults, in their eighties, who maintained frequent sexual activity. In one case, an eighty-six-year-old man had a very large heart attack and was essentially physically limited by his medications and his inability to generate any significant workload. This was due to significant heart damage done at the time of the heart attack. A general rule for a man is that he needs to be able to **easily** climb two flights of stairs with limited symptoms in order to have intercourse. As this man wasn't able to climb even one flight of stairs, he and his wife confided in me that this would be the first time in sixty-five years that they were no longer able to make love every day. Wow! Another seventy-six-year-old man with end-stage heart disease (congestive heart failure) was willing to go off all cardiac medications in order to be able to make love to his "beautiful wife of fifty-five years one last time." These are beautiful and healthy stories of couples who have truly loved each other and enjoyed intercourse together. Of course, as we age there can be a disconnect between what each partner needs from a sexual fulfillment point of view. This is where the comprehensive geriatric assessment excels as the clinicians will often review at sexual health. This is not commonly done in many health care related visits. Sexual activity needs to be fulfilling and safe for both partners. With certain conditions, there are some neurologic processes that can damage our frontal lobe, resulting in hypersexuality or inappropriate sexual behaviour. These concerns need to be openly communicated to the clinician and discussion will occur in a very open manner. Filling out sexual questionnaires is helpful in some situations. A clinician or counsellor can then review the results and address the gaps in sexual desires or other stressors so that the couple understands need for appropriate sexual health and the process is without humiliation, intimidation, or other potentially negative outcomes.

"Sexuality is a core dimension of life that incorporates the notions, beliefs, facts, fantasies, rituals, attitudes, values, and rights with regard to gender identity and role, sexual acts and orientation, and aspects of pleasure, intimacy, and reproduction."[71] There are many entities that influence sexuality. Issues influencing sexuality may include biological, pathophysiological, psychological, social, economic, religious, and spiritual factors. The desire for intimacy is very complex, and this desire for intimacy does not necessary decrease with increasing age.

Sexual health, as with physical health and financial health, isn't simply the presence or absence of sexual function but a state of sexual well-being. There needs to be a positive approach to sexual relationship discussions[72] with the anticipation of a pleasurable experience for both partners. This experience should be without fear, shame, violence, or coercion. While only some clients will discuss sexual dysfunctions with their partners or primary care providers, the attitude of both the partner and the professional has a powerful impact. Opinions and behaviours of sexually active older adult and their comfort in discussing these issues will predict the beneficial impact of those discussion and the state of sexual well being going forward. For every client that has asked a professional for advice regarding their sexual health, there are

---

71 World Health Organization Statement 2008

72 https://pubmed.ncbi.nlm.nih.gov/18637999/

likely many more clients who are too shy or embarrassed to broach the subject. In the comprehensive geriatric assessment, there is a sexual questionnaire called the Personal Assessment of Intimacy in Relationships (PAIR) document. There are other references available on the subject.[73] There are plenty of counsellors available privately to discuss sexuality in more detail should an older adult or couple desire counselling in this important area of life.

A loss of physical and emotional intimacy is profound and often ignored as a source of suffering for the elderly. A transition into assisted living or a nursing home can signal the end of their sexual life. There is a lack of privacy in residential settings, which leads to reduced opportunities for all genders to engage in sexual activities. If clients in care homes are competent to consent to sex and form a relationship, they should be allowed to engage in sexual activities as desired. Some dementia and frontal lobe disease may require a behaviour medicine specialist to be involved, as cognitively impaired older adults have a 1.8 percent prevalence of displaying inappropriate sexual, verbal, or physical behaviour. One of the key points to remember is that the elders are at risk for sexually transmitted infections. Safe sex discussions need to occur at every age group when new partners are meeting.

ASSESSMENTS

If an older adult does need a comprehensive geriatric assessment, the process is lengthy with a multidimensional, holistic assessment of an older person. Many assessments are required by a team of professionals in order to objectively identify the current status of the client. The goal of these assessments is to promote the individual's health and well-being as the top priority. The plan is to address issues that are preferentially, a *concern to the client* (with some input from their family and caregivers if relevant), arrange interventions according to the plan, and review the impact of that plan and then adjust the plan as needed to achieve the goals of the client. This is a prolonged process of which there are many areas to be reviewed including, but not inclusive to:

---

73 Sexuality and Intimacy in Older Adults | National Institute on Aging (nih.gov)

<u>The medical assessment</u> including physical examination, medication review, nutrition assessment, bone health assessment, and pain assessment.

<u>Assessment of functioning</u> includes activities of daily living and instrumental activities of daily living.

<u>Psychological assessment</u> includes cognitive decline, delirium, dementia, and depression.

<u>Social assessment</u> includes social and financial circumstances.

<u>Environmental assessment</u> includes the home visit with allied health professionals including occupation therapists, physiotherapists or other members of the team. Family or friends may also have some insight into whether a client is doing well or not.

<u>Advanced care</u> planning includes the discussion of goals of care for the individual client including rescuscitative efforts, advanced life supporting therapies, substitute decision makers and conditions present which necessitate a change in the plan of care.

<u>Spiritual well-being assessment</u> includes discussions regarding the will to live, the purpose for living, goals not yet achieved and realistic goals to accomplish in the short and long term. These may be religious or non religious based discussions or goals depending on what the client is interested in achieving

<u>Sexuality and intimacy assessment</u> includes the discussion of individual and couple based intimacy goals and discussions to assist with maintaining or improving the quality of life of the individual and couple.

Each of the assessments listed above have readily available guidelines available on the internet. While these have been developed for professional use in health care, the domain site is public and clients or family members can peruse these documents to determine if there is a particular area where the health care team might need to focus on. It's beyond the scope of this book to review the total assessments that can be done. It is important to reiterate, that even one assessment alone may take hours to complete. When done by clinicians familiar with geriatrics or elder care, this truly becomes a comprehensive geriatric assessment due to the time it takes for all the health-care team members to participate and complete their assessments. These assessments are done both in the clinic and the home environment, and acquiring any missing details from family members to fill in the gaps about how the person is really functioning at home is one of the final steps.

Frail older adults are at highest risk of harm when living alone in the general population of older adults. These frail individuals are expected to get the maximum benefit from these comprehensive assessments, but they are often only referred for assessment from the hospital setting. The overall goals of care after these assessments are completed are to:

1. improve physical and cognitive or psychological function
2. optimize medication prescribing and use
3. decrease nursing home placement, hospitalization, and overall mobidity and mortality risk
4. improve patient's satisfaction, which is very desirable, if not the most important goal.

The ultimate goal of the process is to perform an overall assessment, determine the problem list that needs to be worked upon, establish goals of care, personalize the care planning, initiate interventions, and then review the outcomes (positive and negative) in a specified time. Full details can be found at: https://www.cgakit.com/.

CHAPTER SUMMARY

This chapter reviews the concepts of the comprehensive geriatric assessment. Unfortunately, as we all age, most of us won't have access to geriatric specialists. Using the information from the CGA toolkit, clients, families and caregivers can get an overall idea about how they or their loved ones are doing. If primary care access is limited, any time a client is in a hospital or walk-in/urgent care clinic, family should advocate for geriatric assessment to ensure ongoing safety in the home environment.

CHAPTER 16:
THE BUTTERFLY AND THE LOBSTER

It doesn't matter how strong your opinions are. If you don't use your power for positive change, you are indeed part of the problem.
—Coretta Scott King

One of the main concepts in this book is what an individual can do to change the trajectory of their life, so that robustness is maintained, frailty is delayed, falls are prevented, and individuals stay in their comfortable own home until the very end. How can I convince you of how important it is to be interested in these self-help suggestions? How do I make you see the value in the process of actively engaging in these prescribed activity programs? How do I get you to become successful and then boast about the results? I do not have the answers to these questions as yet. I am hoping that you will keep me posted on what motivated you to succeed.

You may not like to exercise. You may feel that losing weight is an exercise in futility. You may feel that they are too old or fragile for exercise. You might believe that arthritis or other underlying conditions will worsen with exercise. But really, there is no reason to avoid increasing your activity level starting today. Even if you do not like change, it is possible to do one small suggestion from this book, even for two minutes and it becomes the start of a new trend.

If you're reading this book, you're clearly wanting to have control of the last third of your life. Reading this book is the first step to helping yourself age in place.

Change is frightening for most human beings. Although change is inevitable at every stage of our development, humans are as not change tolerant as the butterfly. While human beings are not butterflies, and their lifecycle is much different, the butterfly is the master of change management. The adult butterfly is an elder in its last stage of life, and it's beautiful and elegant. The adult lays it eggs before dying. We humans procreate at a much earlier cycle in life. But where I want to focus the attention in this insect analogy, is on some of the parallels of the caterpillar stage, which I feel can be equated to mid and early late life. While the caterpillar does nothing but eat and grow during this stage, humans enjoy a similar period of time in our mid thirties to mid-fifties enjoying life. We don't worry too much about the future during these years. At this stage, we feel that we are invincible, and until our close friends or family members become ill or unexpectedly pass away, we don't really think about our own mortality. And while we are eating, enjoying life, and not looking too far ahead in our future, we have usually succeeded in raising our offspring and are nearing completion of our life's work. We find, in the latter part of these years, that we have some time on our hands that we can use, individually or as couples, to make changes. As I said in an earlier chapter, everyone has to figure out "why" they need to make the changes before those changes will ever come to fruition. At this point, I hope that you have identified the compelling reason for you to take control of your late stages of life now.

The butterfly masterfully enters the pupa stage of change after fattening up. The caterpillar builds a cocoon around itself, and the cocoon is part of its own body. The entire creature begins to liquefy and re-create itself. The butterfly is transforming and grows until it can no longer fit within the cocoon. Its wings eventually poke through the cocoon, and the butterfly erupts as a beautiful, gooey mess. It hangs upside down while its wings dry out, and as we have observed all our lives, this butterfly stage is quite fragile. We can equate this fragile stage to our own stage of life as an elderly person. While humans don't need to lay any more eggs for continuation of the species, this time of our lives is elegantly spent showing the world the true person we have become. The evidence of our fragility, beauty, and strength displayed in our later years. Agism is definitely a trend that unfortunately exists, however, if everyone acknowledged and respected the hard work, survival and wonderful traits of our elderly population, agism would cease to exist. These people have skills that many younger humans will never have, as they have grown up in totally different eras with entirely different skill sets. As a healthcare provider, we need to celebrate the individuality of every senior and help make their final days, weeks, months, or years enjoyable with a quality of life that each individual desires.

Change is difficult! There are times when a person is fully aware that change is required, myself included. Stating the obvious doesn't always help. Good self-esteem is important as we age, and some stubborn individuals (like myself and my father) do not want to be told what to do. As family, friends, and caregivers, we have to try and convey the importance of controlling one's own life, while encouraging and reinforcing positive change. The book is to be used as an instrument to facilitate making change for physical, cognitive, social, and financial health improvements.

Sometimes when change is required, it takes a lot of time to think through what is needed. Every individual brain processes the need for change in a different manner. Some people, like my father, make up their minds and do what they need to do! When my mother broke her hip two years before she passed away, both my parents were two-pack-per-day smokers. They had smoked for sixty-five years each, and my mom was in the hospital getting her hip fixed, without cigarettes. My father, knowing that his wife of sixty years wouldn't be able to smoke anymore, threw his cigarettes away the day she had her hip surgery. He remains a non-smoker today. That was five years ago. I adore these pragmatic folks who just make the required choice happen.

Others need time to process and analyze the benefits of change. These individuals are like the lobster. The lobster in the ocean grows until it is uncomfortable in its current shell. In order to make a new shell, the lobster splits its shell and moves unprotected out of it. It finds an appropriate dark place to hide from predators, usually under a large rock. It stays there until it has grown an entire new exoskeleton. But during this time, the lobster has to lay low, protect itself, and then come up with a game plan once its new shell is made. Many folks are like this. Faced with the need to make changes in life, people can hide and hermit until they figure out their next steps. Sometimes these individuals get "paralysis by analysis," meaning that they continue to analyze the concepts without ever making change.

This is a characteristic of self sabotaging behaviour, and coaching may help these individuals make the changes that are important to them. Coaches can uncover the motivating factors to make transitions more successful so that the individual is able to live their best life.

I have been both the caterpillar and the lobster. As I have done research for this book, I find myself moving into the pupa stage, but I'm not quite at the butterfly stage. By following the game plan that I have laid out in this book, I have lost eighty pounds in the last twelve months. I went through a lot of self reflection on what I needed to do in order to make change, as I had been a caterpillar from age twenty-seven to fifty-eight. I can't tell you how different I feel compared to a year ago with regards to improved energy, improved flexibility, improved endurance, improved strength, improved balance, and improved mood.

CHAPTER 17:
DETERMINING YOUR MOTIVATION FOR CHANGE – KAREN'S STORY

I have grown old too soon and grown smart too late. —Karen's Dad

In this chapter, I will explore the concepts of motivation and coaching for lifestyle change. So far, I have outlined the overall concerns regarding our current health care system, the aging population, the need for more dedicated elder care at the primary care level and at the long-term care/institution level. I have provided some basic education and advice for those attempting to improve their physical and cognitive fitness and functionality, and I have provided some scenarios to consider for financial planning as you age. I mentioned earlier in the book, that the cardio, resistance, and balance exercises are not only recommended by me, but I do them every day. I am not that physician who has been fit and healthy all my life. In fact, for a very long period of time (more than 30 years), I was morbidly obese. When I provide education about how to improve physical and cognitive fitness and functionality, I provide this education fully aware that most people will read this book, find the information helpful on a short-term basis, and then continue with their current habits and way of life. It is my goal to truly make a difference, even in one or two people's lives. However, the scientist in me is fully aware that the literature does not support long-term success in weight loss or even improving fitness levels. In this chapter, I wish to share my story, and I hope by sharing my circumstances, you will successfully find your own reason to make successful and longstanding changes in your lifestyle. For me, it was reflecting on how a very fit young woman ended up with a body-mass index of Grade 3 obesity. I was not successful in changing my lifestyle until I sorted out the reasons that led me to that place and found a most compelling reason to initiate the process of making changes. I expect that for most of you, until you find clarity on the reasons for resisting change in any aspect of your life, change will not occur. In coaching, we call this getting in the way of your own success.

I am five feet four inches tall and have weighed in excess of 100 kg for the last thirty-three years. Before I was married and had children, I was very physically active. Being physically active afforded me the luxury of having a tremendous appetite and love of food, and not having the ill effects of suboptimal body weight or obesity. I was a nurse in health care at a very young age but desired to become a physician. After nursing for several years in the early 1980s, I entered medical school with a four-month-old baby and a less than supportive family network. I commuted six hundred kilometres each week to and from medical school. On the three-hour drive from my home community to Winnipeg, I spent the entire time in my vehicle crying and eating. Many family members and friends led me to believe that I was a bad mother for having career aspirations. I was very stubborn at that time (perhaps I still am as stubborn), and I remember feeling so totally overwhelmed. Even though I had been a registered nurse for many years, my first week of medical school was absolutely gobsmackingly enlightening. As a nurse, with a science degree and a great deal of health care experience, I thought I knew a lot. But in the big scheme of medicine, my knowledge base at that time was a mere drop in a bucket of what I was about to learn, and needed to learn. Then, halfway through my first year of medical school and with a nine-month-old child, I found myself pregnant again. Sadly, the day after I told my ex-husband about the pregnancy, he was involved in a farming accident and lost part of his right hand. I had to immediately quit medical school, and with my tail between my legs, go back to nursing full-time plus overtime to make ends meet for the family. Unfortunately, my ex-husband wasn't eligible for Workers' Compensation or Employment Insurance options due to his unique work situation at the time.

I had gained a lot of weight with my first pregnancy and never lost it. Food was my friend. Food never let me down and improved my mood no matter what was going on in my life. Prior to my first pregnancy, I had the misfortune of having a significant burden of unwanted attention from two men. Of the two men in question, one was a stalker from a past relationship. The stalking did not end until I had married another person and had my first child. I feared this individual for many years. Subconsciously, the unwanted attention went away when I was overweight while pregnant. This became a comfortable scenario, as I felt that I no longer needed to worry about appearances triggering unwanted attention. I became very secure in being overweight and unattractive. It was much safer to exist without the added stress of inappropriate and unwanted attention from anyone. Every hair style and outfit chosen from that time onward reflected my desire to live an anonymous life and not be noted for anything other than my kindness and intelligence.

I went back to medical school the following year, returning with a new four-month-old baby, along with my first child, who was now twenty-two months old. I successfully survived and completed my first and second year of medical school, commuting long distances without my children. The guilt was unbearable. At that time, medical school did not have counselling available for me as I was a unique older medical student. At no point in time do I recall being offered special treatment or any advantage of any kind in medical school. As depression in my ex-husband was becoming more evident, in my third year of medical school, I had to bring my young children to Winnipeg with me. I was a single mother and I needed not only a daycare, but also a private babysitter to look after my children when I was on-call (a necessary and non-negotiable part of medical school training) after usual daycare hours. I had no time to exercise, no time for self-care, and I continued my frumpy single mother look for many years. I didn't want to be perceived as attractive or desirable to any medical student, resident, attending physician, or any other co-worker. I wanted to be "one of the guys" and was considered the older sister of many of my medical school colleagues. I liked it that way. Fast forward to twenty years later, and I was morbidly obese, extremely unhappy, and had depression, but never admitted it due to the stigma associated with mental health disorders in my profession and in the general population. I coped by working excessively (I was a workaholic) and eating anything that was bad for me. This was the stage where I knowingly reflected about how I was killing myself slowly with food. When I wasn't on call, I enjoyed food, wine, and whiskey when I needed to decompress.

In the late winter of 2018, when I had been on call for twenty-seven consecutive twenty-four-hour days in a row, I had an incident at work where I fainted. I was found to be diabetic, which wasn't surprising, as my last baby was delivered before full term and she was very large for the gestational age. My father and my younger sister were also both obese and diabetic.

From 2018 to June 2021, I floundered with my oral medications, injectable insulins, and Semaglutide, and was doing an overall poor job of controlling my blood sugars and my blood pressure. I only went for lab work when I had been a "good diabetic" for two to three months, so I never had a record of an impaired, highly abnormal hemoglobin A1c. I was noncompliant with my regimen, my diet, and any exercise program I attempted. I was the epitome of the non compliant patient, and I really didn't care.

This last paragraph paints a picture of a morbidly obese, depressed, inactive, poorly controlled diabetic with microalbuminuria, hypertension, dyslipidemia, and hypothyroidism. And then, I developed fatty liver disease! The fatigue was overwhelming. Although I had been depressed on and off for many years, in June 2021, the depression became overwhelming.

In March 2019, I lost my mom to metastatic cancer. One of the good things that happened with her death (you need to look for the silver lining in any dark cloud) is that I reconnected with my younger sister, Lisa, and became closer to my dad. Kathy (my older sister), Lisa, and I organized and cleaned out Mother's items as got Dad ready to move to an assisted living home. My younger sister was a poorly controlled diabetic as well. She was on social assistance and lived a marginalized lifestyle. She had always had significant mental health issues even as a young child. She didn't always have a clear understanding of the onset and duration of her insulin therapies and had no idea how to count her carbohydrate intake to dose her insulin correctly. Her glucose was frequently in the 20–30 range, and she was always playing catch-up with her blood sugars. In August 2019, she stayed with me at my house for a weekend. I had an ominous feeling about her health. I talked to her about buying an insurance policy with no evidence, as she wouldn't be considered a candidate for standard life insurance. I felt that both my sister and I would have to go to another province to deal with her final affairs if anything should happen to her, as she was a single woman with no dependents. We talked about making sure she had a will, and for her to start organizing her apartment and getting rid of things she might not need going forward. I think she had a sense as well that her time was limited, as unbeknownst to me, she had left a written statement of what to do with her belongings with my elderly father in our birth province.

On the afternoon of May 24, 2020, I emailed her, as I hadn't heard from her since Mother's Day that year. I thought of her because I suddenly started cleaning out some of the clothes she'd left at my home the prior August, when she was there for the weekend. By ten o'clock that night, I knew she was gone. I didn't sleep all night. I woke up crying in the morning, telling my partner that she was gone. Because she had mental health issues, my partner stated that she could be in a hospital, or she could be gone and time would tell. It was about an hour after this conversation that my father called me to inform me that Lisa had been found passed away in her apartment after many days.

My older sister and I both came from other provinces to clear out her social housing accomodations. We only had four days to go through a very small and crowded apartment. She didn't have a will, the estate was a mess, and the insurance I'd purchased nine months prior wasn't valid because she had to be alive for at least two years before the policy would be in force and pay a benefit. She lived in a marginalized setting with other clients with long standing mental health issues or disabilities. She was socially isolated, and quite frail for her young age of fifty-three. My dad was unable to go and deal with her affairs due to his poor mobility and frailty. My older sister and I looked after everything, but because it was May 2020, and we were in the middle of a global pandemic, we weren't able to say goodbye with a funeral. I really wanted to see my sister's body so I could have some closure. I explained to the funeral director that I was a physician and would likely be okay, as I'd seen many corpses in the past. Her condition at the funeral home precluded any visitation due to the degree of decomposition. She was cremated. She had made it known, prior to her death, that she did not want to be buried in her province of birth. That was her clear wish in that documented, handwritten note left with our father. My sister and I kept her ashes at the funeral home for one year and then decided together, along with our father, that they would come to my home and then be buried with mine when I passed away.

I arranged for my sister's ashes to be returned to me through a courier in mid-May 2021. Her urn sits on one of my bookshelves and looks over me as I work and live, every day. A few weeks after her ashes arrived, I suddenly recognized and accepted what a crappy diabetic patient I had been. I realized that I wasn't taking control of my diet, medications, or exercise. I was socially isolated, or "hermitting," as I call it. I had an appointment with my nurse practitioner for medication renewal. In the first week of June 2021, I had my medications blister-packed, not because I couldn't remember to take them, but I would say, "I'll take them when I'm done (whatever task I was busy with)." Blister packing my medications allowed my partner to easily look at my compliance, and he became my "accountability partner."

I became compliant with taking my oral medications without fail. Within two weeks, I had gone from using approximately sixty units of insulin daily down to twenty-two units a day. Within the next three weeks, I came off insulin completely and had started to become a little bit more physically active. I was certainly much more active in my yard with gardening, but also going for the occasional walk. In mid-June, I purchased a mini stationary bike and kept it in the basement, where I usually watched television. I remember I struggled to do ten minutes on that bike the first week, and today I could bike for several hours while watching a hockey game or football game.

I started losing weight with my SGLT2 inhibitor and metformin, along with limiting my carbohydrates to under 100 g per day and using a caloric intake of 25 kcals per ideal body weight (65 kg). I was still depressed, I acknowledged my depression, and I eventually requested medications for depression. But I had anhedonia, which is when depressed people no longer take pleasure in their usual day-to-day activities. For me, that meant I didn't take pleasure in overeating or indulging in that bowl of icing. And while it did mean that some of my depressive symptoms seemed to be getting worse, and I did require additional medications, after several weeks, some of those medications further assisted with the weight loss. In fact, one of the medications is used for obsessive compulsive disorder, and I was a life long compulsive eater! The other medication is combined usually with naltrexone for obesity management. My medication had the antidepressant alone and not the naltrexone. But I do feel that the combination of depression with anhedonia, medications for depression, and weight loss promoting diabetes medications (empagliflozin and metformin) all contributed to this journey I had attempted to take on my own for over thirty years.

In this last year, I have prioritized my mental and physical health over work. I have figured out why I kept myself obese for many years and have engaged in therapy to work through many longstanding issues. My depression has been treated, and I've lost eighty pounds since June 2021. I do cardio, balance, and resistance training most days of the week. In retrospect, I think that bringing home my younger sister's ashes was the "kick in the pants" I needed to change some of my self-sabotaging habits. I am far from perfect and am still a "work in progress." However, without that kick in the pants, I would still likely be 242 pounds and a poorly controlled, morbidly obese diabetic with severe fatty liver disease!

Exercise prescriptions and cardiac education has been my life's work. Almost forty years ago, I was teaching cardiac care to patients using a vintage carousel slide projector. This was a time before we had any thrombolytic therapy (clot busters) for heart attacks, and patients either succumbed to their heart attacks or became "cardiac cripples." Angioplasty was just becoming mainstream, but unless you were in a large academic centre, the chances of getting this service several hours away was minimal. I worked at a cardiac rehabilitation centre fifteen years ago, and ten years ago I was active in teaching through the Vancouver Island, Heart to Heart cardiac education program, doing evening speaking engagements after clinics to help with cardiac education. I spend my stress testing mornings discussing cardiac rehabilitation and am now incorporating adding in prescriptions for low resistance weight training, balance training, and brain training.

Patients will tell me, "If everyone listened to you, our society would be much healthier." And I would answer, "How do I get people to listen?" This was the impetus for writing this book. I have reflected upon why it took me so long to write a book. The simple answer is, that when I was obese, I had experienced a great deal of fat shaming in my medical professional life. This shaming, destroys one's self esteem. I recalled seeing a specialist for some chest pain I was experiencing a few years ago. I was spoken to in a very a demeaning manner, with him assuming that I knew nothing about cardiac rehabilitation. And yes, this was a thin male about my age, who had never been overweight in his life! With diminished self esteem, I felt that the advice I was giving to patients was not necessarily being taken seriously from the "fat specialist," even though I could relate to the difficulties patients have with lifestyle and medication compliance and the need for weight loss and improved fitness. I did focus a lot on getting patients to buy-in to being a non-smoker first, then a physically fit person second, and achieving ideal body weight was last on those three priorities. Now that I've been successful at following my own advice, I finally feel confident enough to share my life's work with the general public.

Before anyone can change anything in their life, they need to figure out the "why." I have discussed the benefits of these programs in diminishing frailty, in improving physical and cognitive fitness, in aging in place (living in your own home until the end), and having a good quality of life in the later years. But getting depression treated along with the other suggestions in this book will also improve the quality of life and improve the energy required to interact with friends and family.

As it was for me, only *you* can control and change your world.

Now, tell me, what is *your* why? How did you get here, and where do you want to be in one, three, five, or ten years?

CHAPTER 18:
WISH LIST FOR THE FUTURE

No one is in control of your happiness but you; therefore, you have the power to change anything about yourself or your life that you want to change. —Barbara de Angelis

When I talk about the wish list for the future, there are several points that I would like to emphasize.

The first order of business is the fragility of our current health care system and lack of access to primary care. I will elaborate on some of the things I would like to see and what Canadians need to do. The second issue is that of population health and how societies and communities need to push for looking after our population as a whole. Finally, I will elaborate on the concern about the aging population, the current and predicted lack of long-term care home bed access and whether any of these suggestions in the book will promote a more robust aging population.

With regards to our current health care system, there are approximately six million Canadians who do not currently have access to primary care.[74] If Canada was to magically recruit physicians immediately, we would need, today, 3000-6000 new primary care physicians each carrying a patient load of 1000-2000 patients! Canada is expected to be short 44,000 doctors by the year 2028.[75] In addition to this, 33,913 (39%) of the current physicians are older than fifty-five years of age.[76] Canadian medical schools have a quota of admissions at three-thousand per year.[77] Of the approximate 2100 medical students that needed to be trained in a foreign country, only ten percent of those trainees are accepted into Canadian residency programs. There is also a reduced tendency to train in family medicine given the workload

---

74 https://angusreid.org/canada-health-care-family-doctors-shortage/

75 https://thoughtleadership.rbc.com/proof-point-canada-needs-more-doctors-and-fast/

76 https://www.cma.ca/quick-facts-canadas-physicians

77 https://thoughtleadership.rbc.com/proof-point-canada-needs-more-doctors-and-fast/

demands, expensive overhead costs, lack of business training and generational changes in ideology about acceptable work-life balance. In my mind, we can not overcome this massive short coming anytime soon. I believe that we will need to task other members of the health care team to provide team-based care for all Canadians. Where do we get more nurse practitioners, nurses, paramedics, allied health works to fill in the gaps in primary care? There will be competing need to also create and staff more university positions, more long-term care beds and more community clinics. The best advice going forward is that individuals need to start looking after their own health. Secondly, health care needs to use the paucity of professionals currently available and delegate reasonable tasks to other members of the team. This would include certifying more nurses to do pap smears and other certification guided interventions. It may mean paramedics or nurses manage blood pressure monitoring and treatment and refer when algorithms denote a need for a higher level of care. It could also mean using scribes to assist with the unending burden of documentation. Who is the best team member to do well baby care? Preventative screening care? Pap smears? Lifestyle instruction, onboarding and coaching for success? These are just a few of the many tasks in primary care that we as a society need to review and empower our health care leaders to make immediate changes.

The second major issue to fix sooner than later is population health. I do not feel that it is ethical to say we have a functioning health care system, when access is denied to those individuals who can't access emergency health services in a timely manner (ambulance and crowded emergency rooms), can't find any primary care provider and have other concerns in their life related to overall determinants of population health. These folks could also be marginalized, no access to housing, may have food insecurity, abuse and other issues to address.[78] We need a population health strategy and the Government of Canada does acknowledge these concerns. I know many "healthy" adults who are overweight, out of shape, have borderline or high blood pressure

---

78 https://www.canada.ca/en/public-health/services/health-promotion/population-health/population-health-approach/what-population-health-approach.html

(untreated due to lack of access) and could have diabetes, sleep apnea, atrial fibrillation, COPD, cognitive decline or other pathologies that are brewing, but have not yet resulted in a complication. The hospitals are full of folks with heart disease, arrythmias, congestive heart failure, pneumonias, COPD, chronic kidney disease and new onset diabetes triggered or exacerbated by another illness. It is absolutely unacceptable that there is not a robust approach to population health. When I am asked, how do we fix any of this? my answer is truthful. We don't have the human resources to fix anything right now. But if we rely on trying to do the same things over and over again, and expect different results; well, as Einstein put it:

"That is the definition of insanity"

We need to use the resources we have and start small projects in population health while we tackle or primary health care access problem. Health care belongs to Canadians. Let's be sure we are entrusting the right people to make the right changes before it is too late.

In the quote by Barbara de Angelis at the start of the chapter, she was likely referring to happiness in relationships. I find this advice holds true for anything one wants to change. This is an empowering quote for those of us who want to be stronger, wealthier, more fit, weigh less, weigh more, control the rest of one's life and for many other life changes.

My last wish list for the future focuses on the plans proposed in this book.

How are we going to know if any of this will actually work? The first way to make any change is through education. I hope that the concepts in this self-help book have motivated you to try and change the trajectory of your life. If you're deconditioned, out of shape, overweight, diabetic, or have multi-system diseases, you are the answer to your own situation/problem.

For all Canadians with a health concern, I suggest the following:

1. Educate yourself on general cardiovascular risks:
    a. Quit smoking
    b. Get vaccinated
    c. Eat a healthy diet
    d. Limit or abstain from alcohol
    e. Get active (anyway you can)
2. Insure yourself, your life, your employability and the future you:
    a. Financially, we don't know what will happen in the next two decades with health care
        i. Be kind to your family and have life insurance so your remaining family members don't suffer financially while dealing with the worst tragedy of their lives
    b. Insurance applications may (depending on age) result in lab work or other diagnostic tests that may denote an early condition
        i. It is impossible to get lab work done without a primary care provider, unless you apply for insurance above a certain age
    c. Explore options of critical illness insurance for yourself, partners and children
        i. These are not a normal part of company insurance benefits
    d. Explore options for long term care insurance
        i. This is critical is you know you will be a "kinless senior"
3. If you have a sense that there is something wrong, listen to your body:
    a. Check your BP at the pharmacy or buy your own BP machine
        i. Record your readings on a regular basis but don't be obsessive, once or twice a week when well and as needed when feeling poor is sufficient

      ii. Keep track of this and call a nurse's hotline if you are concerned with the readings

b. Check your blood sugar if someone you know has a glucometer, be sure to denote whether you are fasting, pre meal or post meal (1 or 2 hours)

      i. Keep track of this and call a nurse's hotline if you are concerned with the readings

c. If something is not right but you can not decipher if it requires assistance

      i. Go to a walk-in clinic, urgent primary care clinic or call nurse's hotline for advice

      ii. Defer going to the busy emergency room (unless life-threatening or advised to by a professional) if there are other assessment venues available

      iii. Arrange a telehealth appointment and possibly ask for a referral to a local specialist for issues like mental health conditions, systemic illnesses, concerning for underlying malignancy or systemic disease

d. Journal your symptoms, weight and any other unusual things you are noticing

e. Do not ignore sustained palpitations or neurological symptoms

      i. Seek out care in the emergency room if needed

f. Pain that does not go away after a few weeks needs a workup

      i. Contact nurse's hotline, a walkin clinic, an urgent primary care center or an emergency room

      ii. Do not accept narcotics for chronic pain unless there is an indication and a plan for weaning off these medications in less than 4 weeks

g. Concerning symptoms related to heart and lung disease such as activity intolerance, chest pain, shortness of breath, palpitations, cough, sputum production, blood in sputum, vomit, nose, urinary tract or bowels

      i. Present to the Emergency room

Hopefully, after general population education from the above sug-gestions and the book as a whole, we need to hear and share success stories—both personally and system wide.

Clinicians often only hear when things don't go well. All team members are human. Please show your appreciation when someone has gone above and beyond for you or your family. Individually, clinicians often hear about how difficult it is to lose weight as an adult, as only ten percent of people who seek out weight loss are successful in the long-term. But clinicians also need to hear and share your successes with you. While any of the activities in this book may help reduce weight, which is always beneficial, the main point of this program is about preventing falls, frailty, and consequences of frailty through a cardio exercise regimen combined with light resistant training and balance exercise programs. With this, ensuring adequate nutritional intake for our aging bodies is crucial. We need to include adequate amounts of healthy fats, carbohydrates and proteins, and overall calorie and portion-controlled intake, and ideally, complete abstinence from alcohol. We need to create success stories and then share these successes with our friends, family, caregivers, and other social con-nections. There's nothing more motivating than being successful in a goal. All aspects of your physical, mental, and emotional well-being will improve. You'll gain a sense of control over your life and cherish the positive benefits that you and you alone have achieved.

If folks are finding difficulty in improving with this program, it may be due to a physical or mental limitation or undiagnosed condition. Or you may be getting in the way of your own success. Many profes-sionals can provide assistance along the way, including your primary care provider, if you are so fortunate to have one in your life. The role of a life coach is to help you get through your own barriers. There are numerous life and executive coaches available, and I'd recommend that through word-of-mouth references from folks who have had a successful coaching interaction, you seek out those professionals.

With every professional relationship, you must feel safe and trust your professional. If you don't feel comfortable in any way, then look for a new life/business/executive coach. Successful coaching assists you in being the best version of yourself! But this, as in all relationships, is built on trust, requires client accountability, accountability to the coach, and mutual benefit. Some clients are not coachable. Take a hard look at your own circumstances. Are you committed to growing? Are you receptive to coaching/change? Are you open to suggestions, trials of different regimens, or diets? Do you believe what is being said in this book? Will you help others achieve their goals? If you are coachable, then change is possible.

How can we measure success in a community setting? More and more programs are focusing on frailty and identifying, even in primary care settings, scoring systems that result in the identification of clinic clients on the spectrum of frailty (robust to very frail/pre-terminal). There are a lot of new programs looking to address pre-frailty and frailty before interventions such as hip and cardiac surgery. There is a local community effort to try and promote available community programs to address these issues. The United Way in Vancouver has been involved in helping to facilitate social prescribing to limit the loneliness and social isolation the pandemic has unearthed. Caregivers are getting more involved in appropriate medication prescribing and de-prescribing as we age. As a reminder, a lot of the medication studies that were done for many diseases in the last forty years, didn't always include patients over the age of eighty-five. With aging, metabolic processes can alter the way we process medications. We may not have the necessary data to tell a client that what was good for them at seventy years of age is still good at age ninety. We are all living longer, and I'd suggest that medications be reviewed on an annual or semi-annual basis with the prescribers, ideally at age eighty and above.

I would love to see every clinic have a documented list of co-morbid conditions that are part of one of the frailty scoring systems. It is my belief that one of the scoring systems should be used at every clinic and hospital level to track these clients and outcomes. Ideally, a complete medication review would occur with your care providers in client, family, and caregiver team conferences every six to twelve months, and objective assessments that show improvement in one's frailty score, physical state or quality of life are sequentially documented as part of the permanent client record.

With our current primary care crisis, I would like to mention the option of promoting community health centres and population-based care. While we ramp up recruitment and retention for ALL health care team members, I feel that the individual taxpayers, who entrust health care to the governmental authorities, actively promote the concepts of community health centres and population -based care. The CHC concept allows for practitioners to have time off and reduce decrease the incidence of burnout. While there are many advantages to this type of clinic, the major presumption is that CHCs are more costly. What is the cost of quality care? What if CHCs can prevent hospitalization, complications of illness and mortality? Cost benefit ratios will always need to be reviewed with a fiscally responsible government. But we should not WAIT until that data exists. It will be too late.

With regards to population-based care, how many adults have undiagnosed hypertension, diabetes, heart disease, COPD, depression, arrhythmias, thyroid disease, cognitive decline, arthritis, and chronic kidney disease. As a lot of these diseases are asymptomatic, is it right or ethical to ignore those adults without care providers when treatment of an unknown asymptomatic disease, may prevent hospitalizations, complications and death? For me, we need to tackle population-based care now as I stated earlier in this chapter.

Finally, we all have to advocate for better eldercare, which includes the 4Ms of elder care, getting *medications* right, improving *mobility*, enhancing *mentation* (work up and treat delirium, depression, and dementia), and focusing on what *matters*. Advocating for eldercare also includes the need for safe and affordable housing; prevention of emotional, physical, sexual, and financial abuse of elders; increasing social networks/supports with social prescriptions; combating social isolation; and having timely, adequate and reliable personal home support/care services available for the community needs. Seniors also need safe and reliable transportation to and from appointments (for medical, dental, vision, and other basic/critical services and appointments).

Change is difficult for most of us mere mortal human beings. As you look at your life and if you feel powerless about your situation, have faith that you can turn this around yourself. You will require a lot of motivation, a little bit of direction, and you will need to acknowledge and accept the *urgency* of the requirement to prioritize your health *now* before your last twenty years of life fly by.

So, what are you waiting for?

CHAPTER 19:
CONCLUSIONS

In this book, I have elaborated on the three major components required required for successful aging in place. These include but are not limited to adequate fitness and functionality, both from a physical and cognitive perspective, friendly and fruitful family members to facilitate and support safe aging in place and finally, finances to cover the costs of aging when you are no longer willing or able to have regular, employment related money coming into the household.

I have also explored the need for all of us to *identify* frailty, *investigate* for treatable conditions, *initiate interventions that may delay the progression to frailty*, (cardio, resistance training, balance, and brain exercises), *identify* and *improve* care for known chronic conditions that will*inhibit* progression to end stage disease, and evaluate those *interventions* and any *improvements* that have resulted.

In this final chapter, I'd like to explore, what does "aging in place" mean?

When I look at my own family circumstances, I know that my father is very pragmatic and aware of what constitutes quality of life for him at his age. With his permission, my sister and I have had those conversations with our father.

For any family, the elderly client has to figure out these individualized quality of life queries, with the support of the family. For example, here are a few questions to help you derive some of the quality information needed to individualize your "aging in place" plan:

1. What is my reason for living? Do I have my own vision and mission statement? What are my values and goals for the next week, month or year?
2. What key experiences do I want to attempt and have a reasonable chance of achieving?

3. What constitutes an acceptable existence?
4. What are absolutely, the procedures that I DO NOT WANT TO ENDURE under ANY circumstances?
5. Where are acceptable options for accomodations? (Living alone, with without support? Living with family? Institutionalized care?)
6. What are the necessary belongings I need to be with me until the end?
7. How and where do I want to die? (Peacefully at home? With or without family/pets/friends? In hospice care in community? In a hospital?)

The aging in place plan will be different for every individual. The most important concept of the plan is allowing the client to decide what is most important to him/her/them. And while discerning the plan as soon as possible is ideal, the plan will change as health and circumstances change. The good news, is that you still have time to try and delay the frailty portion of aging by choosing not to be frail in the majority of cases. Hopefully, the instructions laid out in the earlier chapters of this book will assist you in achieving this goal.

I have elaborated on a plan to start a slowly progressive exercise regimen that will include a cardio component, a resistance component, a balance component, and a brain component. Some of these components, if done in group settings, will also improve the social interactions that may be missing in your life. There is no right or wrong way to start this program. The most important concept to bear in mind, is that you just need to do something, and then a little bit more each day. While change is incredibly intimidating, anyone at any age, can control how they act and feel with motivation, determination, and a little bit of hard work. As Hippocrates once said, "All parts of the body which have a function, if used in moderation and exercised in labors in which each is accustomed, become thereby healthy, well developed and age more slowly, but if unused, they become liable to disease, defective in growth and age quickly." The bottom line is that if you don't use it, you lose it! This applies to all aspects of one's bodily functions.

If you're considering getting started in order to prevent the complications of falls, frailty, and institutionalization in the future, then I hope you have gathered enough useful information to get the ball rolling. Sometimes accountability is one of the most important factors in predicting success. If you want to become more a more fit version of yourself, meditation and visualization of how you will look and feel as that fit person may assist you. When you have somebody to hold you accountable, it doesn't mean that individual will chastise you if you don't reach your goals immediately. There are supportive coaches and challenging coaches. A mix of both is usually required for success. A friend is somebody who knows the song you're singing and can fill in those words, even when you forget the tune. Friends can act as supportive coaches.

Professionals such as kinesiologists, physiotherapists, trainers, dieticians, and coaches can help with the more challenging aspects of coaching. An accountability partner celebrates your successes as they occur, encourages continued participation when you don't reach your goals as initially set out, supports all of your efforts, and never makes you feel bad at any point on your health journey. Finding that account-ability partner is challenging. Sometimes we don't want anyone else to know how much we weigh or how unfit we are. Fitness, strength, flexibility, balance, and endurance are the goals we as a society need to focus on. At this point in our lives, it's not about dress size or having the same figure as when we were twenty-five years old. This is about improved functionality so that even the most mundane crazy chore, such as having a bowel movement every day, can be done without embarrassment, drama, and trauma.

Society has to stop thinking about and commenting on how anyone looks! You need to start seeking out your accountability partner, as accountability has been one of the key success strategies in programs like Weight Watchers. Once you find that partner and have made the decision that you're going to control your life from here on in, then you have just set yourself up for success. The logistics of coaching and finding that accountability partner includes setting up SMART goals for the client, with accountability and consequences for those goals—specifics of when, where, how long, frequency, responsibility for initiation, and time frame until next reassessment need to be specific, measured, attainable/achievable, relevant, and time sensitive. Congratulations! I look forward to your progress, and please use the attached email address at the end of the book to keep me updated.

Frailty is not an absolute part of aging. There are things we can do in the latter third of our lives to prevent frailty, reduce weakness, and prevent falls. Ultimately the goal is to stay in our own home. Some of us will end up in a personal care home, either because we have no family to safely look after us, don't have the cognition to look after ourselves, don't have the physical capacity to function independently in our activities of daily living, and/or don't have the financial means to afford private or extra care.

Currently, living in long-term care is one of the most dreaded end points that the elderly perceive. However, I can attest to some wonderful institutions that I have worked with over the last four decades. For some seniors, these insitiutions provide a safe place to age and the social interactions prove to be very beneficial both to the individual, their family members, the other residents in the institution and the staff looking after the residents in the home. I have been very fortunate to see some of the best outcomes in my career. That being said, we are entering a time of crisis where access to those very desirable long term care institutions is, and will increasingly be, limited due to our global aging population.

We all have to advocate for better eldercare, better primary care access, better community care supports and more affordable housing and transportation for seniors in our local and national areas. Hopefully, the need for long term careplacement will be delayed for the majority of seniors, so that the limited availability will still be prioritized for those in greatest need and therefore, alleviate some of the pressure on acute care hospital beds. In addition, having the options to chose alternatives in elder care living/accomodation models, (depending on each individual's situation with fitness/functionality, family willingness and availability to assist and innovation/availablility)along with the presence of robust home care services, and financial preparedness should be goals for us all. Most clients want to be independent until the very end or at least dictate what constitutes a quality existence for themselves. We don't want suffering, pain or discomfort. We would prefer in the majority of cases, not to be institutionalized or admitted to hospital. We emphatically prefer not to be a burden on our family members, whom we love dearly. And ideally, we will all die in our own beds, surrounded by our family members or friends or pets, and our death will be peaceful, tolerable, and without drama or trauma for both the patients and their care givers.

As you spring into proactively planning for your own personal fitness and functional journey, I wish you all the best and will be very interested in hearing about your progress.Please feel free to view my website www.kmexecutivecoach.com or email me at mayaandmethuselah2023@gmail.com.

Karen

CONTRIBUTORS, RECOGNITION, AND GRATITUDE

Special thank you to the financial planning consultant:
Mr. Brett McIlwain
Certified Financial Planner®
Victoria, BC
brett.mcilwain.cfp@gmail.com

BIBLIOGRAPHY

Picard, André. Neglected No More: The Urgent Need to Improve the Lives of Canadian Elders in the Wake of a Pandemic. Penguin Random House, March 2021.

Angelou, Maya .And Still I Rise. Random House. 1978

Stall, Nathan. Who Will Care for Canada's Seniors? Ottawa: University of Ottawa Press. 2018 .

Calvin, Sarah. "Geriatric Medicine Profile," Canadian Medical Association Journal 191, no. 5 (2019) E123-125

Canadian Life License Qualification Program. "Life Insurance Essentials Examination." Canadian Life Licence Qualifying Propgram 2015.

Financial Planning Standards Council. "About us." Financial Planning Standards Council , 2023. https://www.fpsc.ca/about us

De Grey, Aubrey "Life Extension Strategies Beyond Calorie Restriction" Nutrition Reviews, 2009.

Canada, Statistics Canada. "Population by sex and age group, by province and territory (2020 Census). "Webpage. Last modified March 28, 2022. Accessed April 21, 2023. https://www150.statcan.gc.ca/n1/pub/82-003-x/2021004/article/00002-eng.htm

Canada, Statistics Canada. "Population by sex and age group, by province and territory (2020 Census). "Webpage. Last modified March 28, 2022. Accessed April 21, 2023. https://www150.statcan.gc.ca/n1/pub/82-003-x/2021004/article/00002-eng.htm

"ECOG Performance Status," ECOG-ACRIN, Cancer Research Group, accessed April 21, 2023, https://ecog-acrin.org/resources/ecog-performance-status.

Canada, Statistic Canada. "Association of Frailty and Pre-frailty with Increased Risk of Mortality among Older Canadians," April 21, 2021, https://www150.statcan.gc.ca/n1/pub/82-003-x/2021004/article/00002-eng.pdf.

"Faster Diagnosis of Frailty in Seniors Aging at Home Is Key to Helping Them Stay Independent," The Conversation, April 7, 2022, https://theconversation.com/faster-diagnosis-of-frailty-in-seniors-aging-at-home-is-key-to-helping-them-stay-independent-177246.

Morley, J.E. and Malstrom, T. K., "A Simple Frailty Questionnaire (FRAIL) Predicts Outcomes in Middle Aged African Americans," National Library of Medicine, July 25, 2015, https://www.ncbi.nlm.nih.gov/pmc/articles/PMC4515112/.

Canada, Statistics Canada. "Association of Frailty and Pre-frailty with Increased Risk of Mortality among Older Canadians," April 21, 2021, https://www150.statcan.gc.ca/n1/pub/82-003-x/2021004/article/00002-eng.pdf.

Evans, W. J. "What Is Sarcopenia?" National Library of Medicine, November 1995, https://pubmed.ncbi.nlm.nih.gov/7493218/.

Government of British Columbia. "Senior Drivers," Government of British Columbia, accessed August 22, 2022, https://www2.gov.bc.ca/gov/content/transportation/driving-and-cycling/roadsafetybc/medical-fitness/seniors

The Dalai Lama XIV. "The Art of Happiness." New York: Riverhead Books. 1998

Canada, Statistics Canada. "Association of Frailty and Pre-frailty with Increased Risk of Mortality among Older Canadians," April 21, 2021. https://www150.statcan.gc.ca/n1/pub/82-003-x/2021004/article/00002-eng.htm

You tube video. "Behind an Accelerated Build: How We Built a Long-term care Home in Ontario in 13 Months." PCL Construction. https://m.youtube.com/watch?v=xpw-diUGOPg

Seniors Advocate BC. (2018). "Quick facts and statistics: Summary report 2018 (PDF file)." https://www.seniorsadvocatebc.ca/app/uploads/sites/4/2018/01/QuickFacts2018-Summary.pdf

Reh-Fit Centre. "Home." Reh-Fit Centre, 2023. https://www.reh-fit.com/

Vieira, Alexandre R. "Pre-test Probabilities and Test Selection in Population Screening and Diagnosis". Journal of Medical Decision Making; March 2020

"How Much Does a Private ECG-Exercise (or Stress) Cost in the UK?" Private Healthcare UK, accessed August 23, 2022, https://www.privatehealth.co.uk/conditions-and-treatments/ecg-exercise-or-stress/costs/.

CBC News. "Ottawa Private Medical Clinic Offers 5-Hour, $1,200 Checkup," CBC, January 15, 2008, https://www.cbc.ca/news/canada/ottawa/ottawa-private-medical-clinic-offers-5-hour-1-200-checkup-1.708173.

CBC News. "Ottawa Private Medical Clinic O"Ottawa Private Medical Clinic Offers 5-Hour, $1,200 Checkup," CBC, January 15, 2008,

https://www.cbc.ca/news/canada/ottawa/ottawa-private-medical-clinic-offers-5-hour-1-200-checkup-1.708173.

False Creek Diagnostics/Wellness. Home page, https://www.falsecreekdiagnostics.com/.

Bennell, Kim L. and Hinman, Rana S. "A Review of the Clinical Evidence for Exercise in Osteoarthritis of the Hip and Knee," accessed August 23, 2022, http://www.yhep.com.au/documents/JSAMS-Article-Osteoarthritis-of-the-hip-and-knee1.pdf.

Allen, Stephen C. "Systemic Inflammation in the Genesis of Frailty and Sarcopenia: An Overview of the Preventative and Therapeutic Role of Exercise and the Potential for Drug Treatments," Geriatrics, January 17, 2017, https://mdpi-res.

com/d_attachment/geriatrics/geriatrics-02-00006/article_deploy/
geriatrics-02-00006.pdf.

Swift, D, and Johannsen, N. et al, "The Role of Exercise and
Physical Activity in Weight Loss and Management," National
Library of Medicine, January 1, 2015, https://www.ncbi.nlm.nih.
gov/pmc/articles/PMC3925973/.

"COPD," Mayo Clinic, accessed August 23, 2022, https://www.
mayoclinic.org/diseases-conditions/copd/symptoms-causes/
syc-20353679.

ATS Ad Hoc Committee on Integretative Medicine.
"Integrative Medicine and the Lung: A New Direction
for the ATS." American Journal of Respirology and
Critical Care Medicine. 189, no. 11 (2014): 1334-
1340. doi:10.1164/rccm.201309-1634ST

ATS Ad Hoc Committee on Integretative Medicine.
"Integrative Medicine and the Lung: A New Direction
for the ATS." American Journal of Respirology and
Critical Care Medicine. 189, no. 11 (2014): 1334-
1340. doi:10.1164/rccm.201309-1634ST

"Lung Function Tests," American Lung Association, accessed
August 23, 2022, https://www.lung.org/lung-health-diseases/
lung-procedures-and-tests/lung-function-tests.

"Pulmonary Rehabilitation," Canadian Lung Association,
accessed August 23, 2022, https://www.lung.ca/research/
pulmonary-rehabilitation.

"Pulse Oximetry," Yale Medicine, accessed August 23,
2022, https://www.yalemedicine.org/conditions/pulse-oximetry.

PCRS-UK, "The mMRC (Modified Medical Research Council)
Dyspnea Scale," accessed April 25, 2023, https://www.pcrs-uk.
org/mrc-dyspnea-scale

Technology for Living Society. "Provincial Respiratory Outreach
Program (PROP)." Technology for Living Society. Accessed

April 25, 2023, https://www.technologyforliving.org/ provincial-respiratory-outreach-program-prop/

Ziglar, Zig. "Secrets of Success." Presentation at Sales and Marketing Conference, Chicago. June 18, 2019

Fragal et al. "RESISTANCE TRAINING FOR OLDER ADULTS: POSITION STATEMENT FORM THE NATIONAL STRENGTH AND CONDITIONING ASSOCIATION." Journal of Strength and Conditioning Research: August 2019-Volume 33-Issue 8-p 2019-2052.

Love Your Age. https://loveyourage.ca/.

Heart and Stroke Foundation. "Could You Use an Exercise Prescription?" Heart&Stroke, accessed August 23, 2022, https://www.heartandstroke.ca/articles/ could-you-use-an-exercise-prescription.

"Diabetes Care Providers Spring into Action," Acadia University, April 25, 2012, https://www2.acadiau.ca/home/news-reader-page/diabetes-care-providers-spring-into-action.html.

Canadian Diabetes Guidelines. https://guidelines.diabetes.ca/ docs/resources/diabetes-and-physical-activity-your-exercise-prescription.pdf.

"Taking Balance Training for Older Adults One Step Further: The Rationale for and a Description of a Proven Balance Training Programme," National Library of Medicine, September 8, 2014, https://pubmed.ncbi.nlm.nih.gov/25200877/.

Bennell, K and Hinman, R. "A Review of the Clinical Evidence for Exercise in Osteoarthritis of the Hip and Knee," accessed August 23, 2022, http://www.yhep.com.au/documents/JSAMS-Article-Osteoarthritis-of-the-hip-and-knee1.pdf.

"14 Exercises for Seniors to Improve Strength and Balance," Lifeline, accessed August 24, 2022, https://www.lifeline.ca/en/ resources/14-exercises-for-seniors-to-improve-strength-and-balance/.

Wall Street Journal. http://online.wsj.com/article/SB10001424052 702304708604577504672437027392.html

"4 Easy Exercises for Seniors Who Are Bedridden," Home Care Assistance, accessed August 24, 2022, https://www.homecareassistanceparkcities.com/ exercises-for-aging-adults-who-are-bedbound/.

Dalia Richmond, "7 Essential Bed Exercises for Elderly," The Geriatric Dietician, accessed August 24, 2022, https://thegeri- atricdietitian.com/bed-exercises-for-elderly/.

Pensions Week. "9 Easy Bed Exercises for the Elderly (and a few to avoid) June 25, 2020. https://www.pensionsweek.com/blog/ bed-exercises-for-elderly

Hugo, Victor (famous French Novelist and poet). "Quotes About Aging." BrainyQuote, accessed April 25, 2023. https://www. brainyquote.com/quotes/victor_hugo_395546.

Robertson, R. Paul and Udler, Mirium S., "Pathogenesis of Type 2 Diabetes Mellitus." Current Diabetic Reports 13, no. 1 (2013): 79-97

Canada Revenue Agency. "Medical Expenses 2023." Canada. ca. Government of Canada. 2023. https://www.canada.ca/en/ revenue-agency/services/tax/individuals/topics/about-your-tax- return/completing-a-tax-return/deductions-credits-expenses/ line -330-other-medical-expenses

D'Agostino, Ralph B, et al, "General Cardiovascular Risk Profile for Use in Primary Care: The Framingham Heart Study," PubMed.gov, January 22, 2008, https://pubmed.ncbi.nlm.nih. gov/18212285/.

Jain, R. et al. "Guideline Endeavor (C-CHANGE) guideline for the prevention and management of cardiovascular disease in primary care: 2022 Update." CMAJ, November 7, 2022; Volume 194, Issue 43 pages E1460-1480. www.cmaj.ca

Canada Revenue Agency. "Medical Expenses 2023." Canada. ca. Government of Canada. 2023. https://www.canada.ca/en/revenue-agency/services/tax/individuals/topics/about-your-tax-return/completing-a-tax-return/deductions-credits-expenses/line -330-other-medical-expenses

Government of British Columbia, "My Voice: Expressing My Wishes for Future Health Care Treatment," accessed August 24, 2022, https://www.health.gov.bc.ca/library/publications/year/2013/MyVoice-AdvanceCarePlanningGuide.pdf.

"One Alcoholic Drink A Day Linked with Reduced Brain Size," PennToday, March 4, 2022, https://penntoday.upenn.edu/news/one-alcoholic-drink-day-linked-reduced-brain-size.

"Ultimate Guide to SMART Goals," AttendanceBot Blog, May 19, 2020, https://www.attendancebot.com/blog/ultimate-guide-smart-goals/.

Canada Revenue Agency. "CPP and OAS Benefits. 2023." Canada. ca. Government of Canada. 2023

Financial Planning Standards Council. "About us." Financial Planning Standards Council , 2023. https://www.fpsc.ca/about us

Financial Planning Standards Council. "About us." Financial Planning Standards Council , 2023. https://www.fpsc.ca/about us62 Government of Canada "A Dementia Strategy for Canada: Together We Aspire,", accessed August 24, 2022, https://www.canada.ca/en/public-health/services/publications/diseases-conditions/dementia-strategy.html.

Men's Health Checklist - Made for Canadian Men (menshealthfoundation.ca)

"NY Times Homepage – Breaking News. US News, World News and Videos."The New York Times. Accessed April 24, 2023. https://www-nytimes-com.cdn.ampproject.org/c/s/www.nytimes.com/2022/12/03/health/elderly-living-alone.amp.html

See Client Reforms from the Financial Industry Regulators (https://www.facsc.ca as an example)

HealthCanada. "Medical Assistance in Dying." Government of Canada. 10 July 2019. https://www.canada.ca/en/health-canada/services/medical-assistance-dying.html

Witt, Scott and Hoyt, Jeff. "Aging in Place – What Does Aging in Place Really Mean?" Updated March 6, 2023. https://www.seniorliving.org/aging-in-place/

OHCHR. (n.d.).About the human rights of older persons. Retrieved April 24, 2023 from https://www.ohchr.org/EN/Issues/OlderPersonPages/OlderPersonsIndex.aspx

Government of Canada. "A Dementia Strategy for Canada: Together We Aspire," Ottawa. Updated February 4, 2019. https://www.canada.ca/en/public-health/services/publications/diseases-conditions/dementia-strategy.html.

World Health Organization. "Sexual and Reproductive Health and Research (SRH)." Statement of Rights. 2008 https://www.who.int

Bitzer, Johannes et al. " Sexual counselling in elderly couples." Journal of Sexual Medicine. 2008 Sep; 5 (9): 2027-2043. Doi:10.1111/j.1743-6109. https://pubmed.ncbi.nlm.nih.gov/18637999/

National Institute on Aging. "Sexuality and Intimacy in Older Adults." nih.gov. Accessed April 24, 2023. https://www.nia.nih.gov/health/sexuality-and-intimacy-older-adults.

Angus Reid Institute. "One in Four Canadians Without Family Doctor, and Access to Care is Uneven, Angus Reid Institute Survey Shows." Angus Reid Institute, 24 Jan. 2019, https://angusreid.org/canada-health-care-family-doctors-shortage/

RBC. "Proof Point: Canada Needs More Doctors and Fast." RBC, 15 Aug. 2019, https://thoughtleadership.rbc.com/proof-point-canada-needs-more-doctors-and-fast/

Canadian Medical Association. "Quick Facts: Canada's Physicians." Canadian Medical Association. Accessed April 24, 2023. https://www.cma.ca/quick-facts-canadas-physicians

RBC. "Proof Point: Canada Needs More Doctors and Fast." RBC, 15 Aug. 2019, https://thoughtleadership.rbc.com/proof-point-canada-needs-more-doctors-and-fast/

Government of Canada. "What is a population health approach?" Public Health Agency of Canada. Updated July 5, 2022. Accessed April 24, 2023. https://www.canada.ca/en/public-health/services/health-promotion/population-health/population-health-approach/what-population-health-approach.html